Nutrition and Dietary Advice in the Pharmacy

Second Ed

PAMELA MASON
BSc(Pharm), MSc, PhD, MRPharmS

**Blackwell
Science**

© 1994, 2000 by
Blackwell Science Ltd
Editorial Offices:
Osney Mead, Oxford OX2 0EL
25 John Street, London WC1N 2BL
23 Ainslie Place, Edinburgh EH3 6AJ
350 Main Street, Malden
  MA 02148 5018, USA
54 University Street, Carlton
  Victoria 3053, Australia
10, rue Casimir Delavigne
  75006 Paris, France

Other Editorial Offices:

Blackwell Wissenschafts-Verlag GmbH
Kurfürstendamm 57
10707 Berlin, Germany

Blackwell Science KK
MG Kodenmacho Building
7–10 Kodenmacho Nihombashi
Chuo-ku, Tokyo 104, Japan

First published 1994
Reprinted 1997, 1998 (twice)
Second edition 2000

Set in 10/12pt Sabon
by DP Photosetting, Aylesbury, Bucks
Printed and bound in Great Britain by
The Alden Press, Northampton and Oxford

1001926210

DISTRIBUTORS

Marston Book Services Ltd
PO Box 269
Abingdon
Oxon OX14 4YN
(*Orders:* Tel: 01235 465500
        Fax: 01235 465555)

USA
Blackwell Science, Inc.
Commerce Place
350 Main Street
Malden, MA 02148 5018
(*Orders:* Tel: 800 759 6102
        781 388 8250
        Fax: 781 388 8255)

Canada
Login Brothers Book Company
324 Saulteaux Crescent
Winnipeg, Manitoba R3J 3T2
(*Orders:* Tel: 204 837 2987
        Fax: 204 837 3116)

Australia
Blackwell Science Pty Ltd
54 University Street
Carlton, Victoria 3053
(*Orders:* Tel: 03 9347 0300
        Fax: 03 9347 5001)

A catalogue record for this title is available
from the British Library

ISBN 0-632-05368-2

Library of Congress
Cataloging-in-Publication Data
Mason, Pamela.
    Nutrition and dietary advice in the pharmacy/
Pamela Mason.—2nd ed.
        p. cm.
    Includes bibliographical references and index.
    ISBN 0-632-05368-2 (pb : alk. paper)
    1. Nutrition counseling.   2 Diet therapy.
  3. Pharmacists.   I. Title.
    [DNLM: 1. Diet Therapy.   2. Diet.
  3. Nutritional Requirements.   4. Pharmacists.
  WB 400 M4115n 2000]
  RM 218.7.M37 2000
  613.2—dc21
                                99-088944

For further information on
Blackwell Science, visit our website:
www.blackwell-science.com

Contents

Preface to the First Edition

As a community pharmacist running my own business some years ago, I became convinced that the potential for pharmacists to give nutritional advice is enormous. Postgraduate study in nutrition at King's College in London increased this conviction and supplied much of the background knowledge which has enabled me to write this book.

Interest in nutrition continues to grow but much of the information received by the public is sensational and unbalanced, creating confusion and uncertainty. The need for accurate and unbiased advice is undeniable, and as a pharmacist you are well placed to provide it.

Your position at the forefront of community health care means that dietary advice can reach members of the public who are not necessarily in contact with dietitians or other health professionals. Many people visiting pharmacies are relatively healthy, and you can make a unique contribution to the promotion of healthy eating and prevention of disease in later life.

Diet plays a crucial role in the management of several conditions, such as diabetes mellitus and coeliac disease. After initial diagnosis, patients may not see the dietitian or GP regularly, but they do go to pharmacies. Dietary changes can be difficult to make, and patients value consistent and informed support.

I have sought to address the many opportunities for giving dietary advice which you are likely to encounter in a community pharmacy, and this book will help you to:

- offer practical advice on healthy eating and food safety
- confirm the importance of diet in the management of conditions such as hyperlipidaemias, hypertension, diabetes mellitus and coeliac disease
- recognise the need for the professional advice of a dietitian and refer patients when necessary
- give appropriate nutritional advice with products commonly sold in the pharmacy, e.g. slimming products, infant milks, baby foods and dietary supplements
- recognise the nutritional needs of specific groups of people including pregnant women, the elderly, athletes and cultural minorities
- advise patients on food and diet in connection with their prescribed medication
- give encouragement and support to patients who are maintained on enteral and parenteral nutrition at home

It is my hope that pharmacists will be recognised as providers of sound nutritional advice in the community. This book is an attempt to help them fulfil this role.

I would like to acknowledge the advice and support of a wide range of people, including colleagues working on the British National Formulary and those at the National Pharmaceutical Association. Particular thanks are due to Mrs Brenda Ecclestone and Miss Joan Mason for reading the manuscript and making valuable comments, and also to my husband Ambrose for the encouragement and support he has given me throughout the writing of this book.

Pamela Mason

Preface to the Second Edition

Since the first edition of this book was published in 1993, there have been a number of important changes in the field of food and nutrition. Recent research has pointed to the importance of several new dietary links in cardiovascular disease, notably folic acid; other factors such as phyto-oestrogens and bioflavonoids are beginning to emerge, not only as protective factors in cardiovascular disease, but also in cancer. The incidence of over-weight and obesity continues to increase, making advice on weight control ever more important for people of all ages including children and adolescents. Each chapter has been updated to include these and a number of other changes.

What has not changed since the first edition, however, is the need for dietary advice and the opportunity for pharmacists to provide it. Individuals are increasingly interested in diet as a means of maintaining and improving their health, although public scepticism has increased as a result of recent food scares such as BSE and salmonella. With the internet, the amount of nutritional information available to the public is growing enormously; an easily accessible and well-informed health professional can help to make sense of this.

A number of readers have been kind enough to make the effort to make comments on the first edition, and I have tried to act on their suggestions. I would be grateful to receive further comments in the future.

Section 1
Communication of Dietary Advice

Chapter 1
The Role of the Pharmacist

Introduction

Nutrition is an area of growing interest to the public. During recent years we have all been bombarded with information about diet from the media (including the Internet), advertisements and food manufacturers. Some of this information is reliable but some is not and most people do not know the difference.

A source of sound, unbiased dietary advice is therefore essential, and pharmacists are well placed to provide it. Although dietitians are the experts in this field, there are currently too few of them in community practice to give individual dietary advice to all those who need it. Community pharmacists are much more accessible.

Many customers in community pharmacies are relatively healthy. This makes the pharmacy an ideal place for providing information and advice to prevent illness, and promote healthy eating. Dietary advice can reach members of the public who are not necessarily in contact with dietitians or other health professionals.

Why is dietary advice important?

The importance of good diet has been known for a long time. The discovery of vitamins in the early 1900s confirmed the belief that a wide variety of foods was important for growth in children and for maintenance of health in adults. This knowledge was transferred into medical practice and national nutrition programmes. Dietary advice emphasised the importance of meat, fish, cheese, eggs, milk, and fruit and vegetables as the best sources of essential nutrients, and as the variety and quality of food improved the number of people diagnosed with overt nutritional deficiencies fell.

After the Second World War, medical practice was dominated by the power of antibiotics and other drugs, and emphasis on dietary advice declined. At the same time food patterns also changed; in general there has been a reduction in cereal and root vegetable intake and a steady increase in the consumption of animal products. This has led to an increase in the consumption of fat, particularly saturated fat, and a fall in starchy carbohydrate.

By the 1960s evidence was emerging that diseases not normally associated with malnutrition were linked with diet. Nutritional concepts began to change as research showed links between nutritional excesses, as well as deficiencies, and the development of such diverse conditions as coronary heart disease, cancer and gallstones.

Although incomplete, research findings linking diet to disease are sufficiently convincing for many government committees to recommend changes in national diets. In 1991 the UK Department of Health's report *Dietary Reference Values for Food, Energy and Nutrients for the United Kingdom* made several dietary recommendations. These included a reduction in the average proportion of food energy derived from total fat and saturated fatty acids, a reduction in sugar and an increase in dietary fibre. These recommendations have been reiterated in many publications since that time and have been incorporated into the UK's National Food Guide.

Achievement of such targets requires more than exhorting individuals to make dietary changes; changes in social and economic policy are also crucial to allow people to choose a healthy diet. Nevertheless, by providing sound dietary advice, pharmacists can make an important contribution to the achievement of these targets.

Opportunities for the pharmacist

Pharmacists have many opportunities to provide nutritional information, but they should always be aware of their limitations and know when to refer a person to a dietitian. In the first instance this will usually mean a referral to a GP.

As an integral part of pharmaceutical care, dietary advice may be appropriate with prescription and over-the-counter medicines, when responding to symptoms, and with products supplied in the pharmacy which have nutritional implications. Pharmacists offering screening services have further opportunities for giving dietary advice.

Medicines

Pharmacists will certainly be used to advising patients about the timing of medicine administration in relation to food intake, but drugs interact with nutrition in several ways (see Chapter 26). Drugs may induce vitamin and mineral deficiencies, alter taste and appetite or lead to changes in body weight. On the other hand, vitamin and mineral supplements may lead to changes in drug absorption and metabolism, and pharmacists will be aware that many drugs interact with alcohol. Pharmacists should be aware of such interactions and be prepared to counsel the patient or discuss a change of drug with the prescriber.

Consideration should also be given to the disease for which the drug has been prescribed. A patient taking an oral hypoglycaemic drug such as glibenclamide does not need to be given any specific dietary advice as far as the drug is concerned. However, a person with diabetes might value some advice and encouragement on losing weight or controlling fat and sugar intake.

Initial dietary advice in disease states will be given by a dietitian, but the pharmacist should have sufficient knowledge and understanding to encourage the patient to persevere with any recommended dietary change. (See Section 3 for the role of diet in the management of disease.)

Responding to symptoms

When asked for advice about symptoms, dietary advice could be more appropriate than supplying a medicine. For example, a person with constipation would be better advised to eat more wholemeal bread and wholegrain cereals than buy a laxative.

Products with nutritional implications

Pharmacists supply many products which have nutritional implications. Dietary advice may be appropriate with gluten-free foods (see Chapter 9), infant formula milks and baby foods (see Chapter 16), slimming products (see Chapter 19), dietary supplements (see Chapter 25) and enteral and parenteral feeds (see Chapters 28 and 29).

Screening

Screening services such as measurement of blood pressure, body weight or serum cholesterol often provide an opportunity for giving dietary advice.

People buying pregnancy or ovulation kits will also benefit from dietary advice if they are pregnant or planning to become so. Patients with diabetes can be reminded about the importance of diet when they buy blood and urine glucose testing kits.

Dietary advice

Pharmacists must give dietary advice which is accurate, consistent and up to date. There is a great deal of conflicting nutritional information around, and pharmacists should be able to interpret such information objectively and correct any misconceptions. This demands a sound and up-to-date knowledge of nutrition.

Giving dietary advice means more than just telling a person what to eat. Consideration must first be given to the individual's background and personal circumstances and other factors which may affect food choice. Pharmacists need to recognise that other people's knowledge and beliefs about food may be very different from their own.

What influences food choice?

An understanding of the factors affecting food choice is important because they are likely to affect a person's ability to make changes to their diet. Fig. 1.1 illustrates some of these factors.

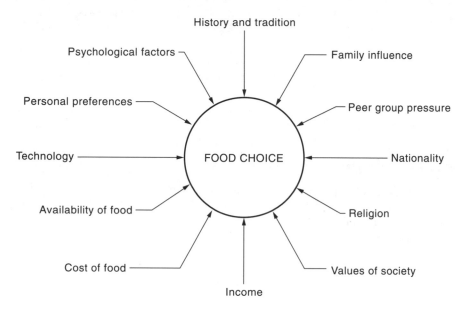

Fig. 1.1   Factors affecting food choice.

History and tradition

Throughout the world, eating habits are governed by history and tradition. Before the industrial revolution the majority of British people consumed a diet based on coarse bread, cheese, eggs, ale, fish and sometimes meat with a few vegetables. Wealthy people ate more luxuriously and included generous amounts of meat, fruit and vegetables in their diet.

At the time of the industrial revolution many people went to live in the towns so food had to be transported from the countryside. Improvements in farming methods and international trade provided urban populations with increased quantities of meat, milk, dairy products, fresh fruit and vegetables. Tinned food became available for the first time in 1880. After the First World War the government gave greater priority to food production with special emphasis on meat and dairy products because such foods were considered to be the basis of a good diet.

It is not surprising that people are confused and somewhat resistant to dietary advice which now advocates a return to a diet based on grains with smaller amounts of meat and dairy produce.

Culture

Food selection is learned from an early age. Childhood experiences have a strong influence on the foods people choose in later life. Peer group pressure can have a strong influence on food choice in older children. It can be hard to persuade children to keep off sweets if that is what their friends are eating.

Other cultural influences on food choice include religious beliefs and nationality. Hindus do not eat beef and Muslims avoid pork. People from many different countries have come to live in the UK and continue to follow traditional dietary patterns to varying degrees (see Chapter 23).

Travel abroad has encouraged many people to try traditional dishes from other countries and these foods are becoming increasingly popular in the UK. What were once exotic fruits and vegetables are now easily available and most of us take for granted the ability to buy pasta, basmati rice, taramasalata, poppadoms, bean sprouts, water chestnuts and a wide variety of dried pulses.

The values held by society at any one time may affect people's food choice. For many the advice to increase consumption of wholemeal bread and wholegrain cereals is entirely consistent with a popular desire to return to a 'natural' way of life. Yet for others meat is a status symbol which their grandparents treasured as a treat and could ill afford.

Availability

Availability is one of the most important determinants of food choice. While large supermarkets stock a wide variety of foods, many small shops stock a much more limited range. In giving dietary advice pharmacists should be aware of the types of shop their customers can get to and what is available in them.

Economics

People's food choice may be limited by their income (see Chapter 24), and sensitivity towards people's financial circumstances is important. While a healthy diet need cost no more than an unhealthy one, it may still be beyond the means of poorer people. Suggestions to increase consumption of fruit and lean meat can seem prohibitive to an individual trying to feed a large family on a small income. Less healthy choices of food such as sausages, pies, biscuits and cakes are much cheaper. Even wholemeal bread is more expensive than white bread.

Food preparation

Refrigerators, freezers, microwave ovens and food processors have considerably widened people's choice of meals. Time is also an important factor in food preparation, particularly for the increasing numbers of women who go out to work and continue to be the main providers of food in the home. Although there is a large variety of take-away and convenience foods, these are not always either nutritionally sound or cheap.

Psychological factors

One of the most obvious factors affecting food choice is personal preference. Although this can change with time, people will only eat what they enjoy.

Sweet foods are often used as a reward during childhood and may continue to be viewed as treats in adulthood. Compulsive eating is often a way of fighting depression, boredom and loneliness.

Giving dietary advice

Giving dietary advice means starting where the person is at. Advice which takes no account of lifestyle and personal circumstances is bound to fail. If business lunches are a regular occurrence, dietary advice must take account of this.

It is important to ask questions about current dietary habits. There is certainly a need to recognise that some people will already have improved their eating habits and it is pointless advising an increase in fibre intake if the person already eats wholemeal bread with every meal.

The very precise dietary advice which dietitians are qualified to give depends on obtaining an accurate dietary history from the patient, and calculating nutrient intake from food tables. Few pharmacists would have the time, expertise or resources to do this, but some attempt should be made to assess current eating habits. The best way of approaching this is by sensitive discussion rather than by a lot of point-blank questions which may well make the person feel intimidated.

As a starting point the quantity of fruit, vegetables, bread and cereals consumed should be established as well as the type of spreading fat and dairy products used. Cooking methods and the frequency of consumption of fatty and sugary snacks should be discussed. A quick comparison can then be made with the practical dietary guidelines discussed in Chapter 3.

Once a person's lifestyle and eating habits have been established, the pharmacist can give general guidance on the direction in which the diet needs to be changed. Some people may need to make small changes to their diets, but others will need guidance making more significant and difficult adjustments.

All dietary advice must be realistic and must not depart dramatically from the person's existing habits. Individuals must have the money, time and facilities to buy and prepare the necessary foods. Although dried pulses are cheap and healthy, they are time consuming to prepare; canned pulses are just as healthy and although more expensive they are certainly more convenient.

It is unreasonable to expect people to follow dietary advice without an explanation of why such changes are necessary. Many people who need to make changes to their diet have no symptoms of disease, and however careful the instruction it may be unsuccessful if the reason for it is not understood.

Dietary advice should always be positive; the 'stop eating' approach is negative and unlikely to be successful. For too long dietary advice has been synonymous with dietary restriction so foods of which people ought to be eating more such as bread and fruit should be mentioned first and given special emphasis. If a particular component of the diet is to be reduced, advice should always be offered on possible replacements.

One common misconception is that there are 'good' and 'bad' foods. In reality there are only good and bad diets. In fact it is probably better to avoid the words 'bad' and 'good' altogether when talking about diet; healthy and unhealthy are preferable terms. The inclusion of an occasional bar of chocolate or a packet of crisps cannot by itself ruin an otherwise satisfactory diet. It is only when these foods are consumed in large quantities that the diet may be considered to be unhealthy. Conversely, eating an apple every day will do little to improve an unhealthy diet unless healthy choices are made from other foods as well.

Dietary advice should always be specific. Many people know that they should reduce their fat and sugar intake, but not how to go about it because they do not know which foods are high and low in fat and sugar. It is all very well telling people to increase or reduce a component of their diet, but by how much? Which foods should they be eating and in what sort of quantities?

People often find dietary changes difficult to make so too many changes should not be recommended at once. People used to the taste of full cream milk often find the taste of fully skimmed milk detestable, but they could probably be persuaded to try semi-skimmed milk at first.

In any case, people tend not to be able to remember more than three or four pieces of information at once so that advice should be as brief and as clear as possible. Dietary advice should always be free of jargon, and an attempt should be made to use language the person will understand without being patronising.

The pharmacist should agree a plan of action for dietary change with the person and not just tell them what to eat. The individual should be encouraged to comment and ask questions to make sure that the dietary advice has been understood. Leaflets can be useful as a means of reinforcing this but should not be used as a substitute. People should also be encouraged to return for follow-up or to seek more information if they feel they need it. Pharmacists should be aware of other sources of nutrition information, and in some cases this may mean referral to a dietitian.

Motivation and compliance

Even with the most careful instruction people tend to be very resistant to making dietary changes. Risk of disease at some unknown point in the future is not always a sufficient motivating force. Even when illness has been diagnosed, people do not always comply with dietary advice. People with diabetes often find it extremely difficult to lose weight even though by so doing they might not need to take hypoglycaemic drugs.

Healthy eating must be enjoyable. Memories of soggy cabbage from school lunch days may discourage vegetable consumption, and creative methods of cooking and presentation are needed to encourage people to eat them. Most people know that they should reduce their fat intake, but if they live in a household where everybody likes chips, it may be very difficult.

Communication of dietary advice is summarised below:

> (1)   Start with the individual; establish background, personal circum-stances, lifestyle and beliefs about nutrition
> (2)   Establish current eating habits
> (3)   Explore willingness and possibilities for dietary change
> (4)   Agree three or four (no more) dietary changes with the individual
> (5)   Offer follow-up and/or advise about other sources of information
> (6)   Refer to a dietitian if necessary (through the GP)

Further reading

Williams, D. (1997) *Communication Skills in Practice. A Practical Guide for Health Professionals.* Jessica Kingsley Publishers, London.

Section 2
Diet in Health

Chapter 2
Dietary Guidelines

The fact that a balanced diet provides all the essential nutrients is well known. But what is a balanced diet? The concept of balance has arisen from a concern that the diet should provide sufficient amounts of all the essential nutrients to prevent the development of deficiency diseases such as scurvy. Now that the prevalence of overt deficiency disorders has decreased, the term 'balanced diet' is less appropriate.

The present need is to alter the proportions of food items consumed (e.g. fats and carbohydrates) and, at the same time, to ensure an adequate intake of essential nutrients. The term 'healthy diet' is now considered to be more useful than 'balanced diet' and will be used throughout this book.

But what is a healthy diet? This can only be answered if there are standards against which people's nutrient intakes can be measured.

Dietary standards

Until recently, dietary standards in the UK existed in the form of Recommended Intakes for Nutrients (DHSS 1969) and Recommended Daily Amounts (RDA) of food energy and nutrients (DHSS 1979). These were designed to ensure an adequate intake of energy and essential nutrients including protein, vitamins and minerals.

These standards were often misused. The RDA was often interpreted as the minimum desirable intake for optimal health and an amount which everybody had to consume. In reality, the RDA is normally in excess of what most people need – at least to prevent deficiency. In addition, they were often used to assess the diets of individuals when they were intended to be used for groups of people, and a greater degree of accuracy was attributed to them than was intended.

More recently the adverse effects of excessive consumption of nutrients, in particular fats, have received attention, and dietary standards have evolved from their original use in the prevention of deficiency disease to their current use in the maintenance of good health.

The most recent dietary standards in the UK (DOH 1991a) have been developed in the form of Dietary Reference Values (DRVs) which can be found in Appendix 1. They combined guidance for intakes of essential nutrients to prevent deficiency as well as proportions of fats and carbohydrates which should contribute to the prevention of chronic degenerative disease. However, DRVs do not currently provide guidance on intakes of vitamins and minerals which might help to reduce the risk of conditions such as cardiovascular disease and cancer.

DRVs, like RDAs, should only be used to assess the diets of groups of people rather than individuals, and they are guidelines for reference rather than recommendations. DRVs are not designed for patients with disease, some of whom may have different needs from those of healthy people. Despite these caveats DRVs do serve as a useful guideline for judging the adequacy of an individual's diet.

Standards for energy, protein, vitamins and minerals

DRVs for energy, protein, vitamins and minerals are defined in broad age classes and separately for pregnancy and lactation (see Appendix 1).

Deciding how much energy a person requires to maintain ideal body weight or how much protein, vitamin A or iron is needed for optimal health is difficult for many reasons. This is because people differ from each other in the amounts of energy and nutrients they need. Energy and nutrient needs depend on age, sex, physiological status (e.g. pregnancy) and the presence of disease. A further difficulty is that nutrient absorption varies; this depends not only on need (i.e. the level of the body stores) but also on factors such as the presence of other dietary constituents or drugs in the intestines.

The information used to set dietary standards includes:

- The intake of a nutrient needed to prevent or cure symptoms of deficiency
- The intake of a nutrient required to maintain a given blood or tissue concentration or degree of enzyme saturation
- The intake of a nutrient required to maintain balance (i.e. intake – output = zero)
- Food and nutrient supplies of healthy populations

The requirements for a nutrient in a group of individuals is assumed to follow a normal distribution curve (see Fig. 2.1). The RDA was set at 2 standard deviations above the mean requirement and designed to cover the needs of 95% of the population, even those with high intakes. To overcome the potential for misuse with this single figure (the RDA), a set of figures has now been developed (see Table 2.1). These include the Estimated Average Requirement (EAR) or mean requirement, the Reference Nutrient Intake (RNI) which, like the old RDA, is defined as 2 standard deviations above the EAR, and the Lower Reference Nutrient Intake (LRNI), which is defined as 2 standard deviations below the EAR.

Standards for fat and carbohydrates

Fats and carbohydrates differ from protein, vitamins and minerals in that, with the exception of essential fatty acids, there are no symptoms of

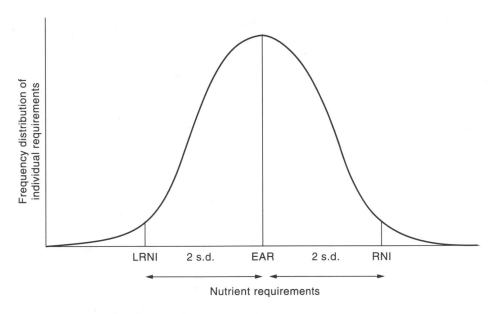

Fig. 2.1   Frequency distribution of nutrient requirements.

deficiency associated with low intakes and no absolute requirements. However, the proportions of fat and carbohydrates in the diet may influence health, and DRVs have been set which are considered to reduce the risk of development of chronic degenerative diseases such as coronary heart disease and cancer.

Establishing the evidence

Proof of cause and effect relationships in studies of diet and chronic degenerative disease is extremely difficult to obtain. While it is easy to show that a deficiency of vitamin C causes scurvy, it is virtually impossible to prove that a single component of diet causes cancer. Chronic degenerative disease is, in any case, multifactorial, and environmental and genetic factors play an important part.

Dietary factors currently associated with some diseases are summarised in Table 2.2, but as research proceeds the relative importance of risk factors is likely to change.

Some of the difficulty in establishing causation is that chronic degenerative diseases tend to develop over many years and the disease could be the result of long exposure to specific components of diet. It is difficult to assess dietary intake over such a long period because people find it difficult to remember what they have eaten. Investigations of current food intake provide limited information because current dietary patterns do not necessarily reflect past intake.

Table 2.1   Definitions of dietary standards.

DRV	Dietary Reference Value. A term used to cover LRNI, EAR, RNI and safe intake
EAR	Estimated Average Requirement. An assessment of the average requirement for energy or protein or a vitamin or mineral. About half the population will need more than the EAR, and half less
LRNI	Lower Reference Nutrient Intake. The amount of protein, vitamin or mineral which is considered to be sufficient for the few people in a group who have low needs. Most people will need more than the LRNI, and if people consistently consume less they may be at risk of deficiency of that nutrient
RNI	Reference Nutrient Intake. The amount of protein, vitamin or mineral which is sufficient for almost every individual. This level of intake is much higher than many people need
Safe Intake	A term used to indicate intake or range of intakes of a nutrient for which there is not enough information to estimate RNI, EAR or LRNI. It is considered to be adequate for almost everyone's needs but not large enough to cause undesirable effects
RDA	Recommended Daily Amount. The average amount of energy or a nutrient recommended to cover the needs of groups of healthy people

The evidence relating diet to chronic diseases comes from several types of study. These epidemiological investigations include case–control studies, cohort studies and controlled trials. In addition, the techniques of meta-analysis and pooled analysis have been developed to provide summaries of selected collections of studies.

Epidemiological investigations

Epidemiological investigations look at different populations and the associations between dietary factors and chronic diseases. The most consistent correlations have been obtained from studies of populations or population subgroups which have substantially different dietary habits. For example, until recently the Japanese have had a low fat diet and a low rate of heart disease. Americans – although they are changing now – have consumed a high fat diet and have had high rates of heart disease. Japanese people living in Hawaii, with an American lifestyle, eat more fat and have more heart disease than Japanese people living in Japan. But it is important to realise that there are anomalies in the epidemiological data. Fat intake in France, for example, is just as high as in Britain yet the French have much lower rates of coronary heart disease. Generous wine consumption may contribute to the relatively low rates of heart disease in France by reducing the clottability of the blood.

One of the problems with epidemiological studies is that at best they can only be used to predict disease rates for large groups of people. In other words, they examine the 'big picture'. In contrast, it is much more difficult to

Table 2.2 Associations between dietary components and disease.

Disease	Body wt	Fat	Saturated fat	Fibre	Sugar	Salt	Alcohol	Ca	Fruit and vegetables	Smoked, salted and pickled foods
CHD	+	++	++	–		+	+/–		–	
Hypertension	++	+	+			++	+	–		
Cancer										
Stomach									–	++
Rectum		+	+						–	
Liver							+		–	
Lung										
Breast	+	+	+							
Endometrium	++	+								
Prostate	+	+	+							
Obesity		+		–	+		+			
NIDDM	++									
Constipation				–						
Haemorrhoids				–						
Gallstones	++			–						
Dental caries					+					
Osteoporosis	–						+	–		

+ Weak positive association; ++ strong positive association; – negative association; CHD, coronary heart disease; NIDDM, non-insulin dependent diabetes mellitus. (Adapted from *Diet, Nutrition, and the Prevention of Chronic Disease*, WHO 1990.)

identify an association between disease and diet within one population or country where the diets of individuals are fairly similar.

Case–control studies

Many of the weaknesses of epidemiological investigations can be avoided in case–control studies, in which patients with a specific disease (the cases) and a comparable group of people without the disease (the controls) are identified from the same source population. Information is obtained from each case and each control about their earlier diet. It may then become evident that the cases report (say) higher levels of fat intake than the controls. Although case–control studies reduce many of the confounding factors evident in larger epidemiological studies, one of their difficulties is that individuals may misrepresent past diets.

Cohort studies

In prospective cohort studies, the diets of a large group of healthy individuals are followed – usually for 10 years or more – during which a number of people will develop the disease in question. The relationship between the disease and specific characteristics of the diet is then analysed.

Controlled trials

Controlled trials use a control group of people given an inactive substance, and an intervention group given a dietary component which may influence disease risk. The preferred method is the 'randomised controlled trial' in which people are assigned to an intervention group at random.

The problem with intervention studies looking at aspects of diet and disease is that it takes such a long time for the risk of chronic disease to become evident. It is also extremely difficult to obtain reliable information and people's diets over a long period of time.

Use and abuse of the evidence

The evidence for links between diet and disease has been established for whole populations, but there is often much less support for such associations at the individual level. Pharmacists, however, deal with individuals rather than groups of people, and what individuals want to know is whether they personally are going to die of a particular disease if they do not make the suggested dietary changes. Unfortunately, it is often difficult to say.

Individuals should never be misled into believing that adherence to some specific recommendation will ensure avoidance of chronic disease. On the other hand, failure to follow dietary guidelines does not necessarily mean that the individual is doomed to an early death. What can be expected is that if the whole population adopts the recommended dietary pattern, the incidence of chronic disease will decline. For individuals it is only possible to talk in terms of reducing risks and improving chances; there are no absolute certainties. However, as more becomes known about individual biochemistry and the influence of nutrients on that it may, within a few years, be possible to give individuals more precise nutritional advice.

Current healthy eating guidelines provide the basis for the choice of a healthy diet which incorporates current knowledge and which is likely to prevent nutritional deficiency and reduce the incidence of chronic disease in the population.

Further reading

DHSS (1969) Recommended intakes of nutrients for the United Kingdom. Report on Public Health and Medical Subjects No 120. HMSO, London.

DHSS (1979) Recommended daily amounts of food energy and nutrients for groups of people in the United Kingdom. Report on Health and Social Subjects No 15. HMSO, London.

DOH (1991a) Dietary reference values for food energy and nutrients for the United Kingdom. Report on Health and Social Subjects No 41. HMSO, London.

DOH (1991b) *Dietary Reference Values. A Guide.* HMSO, London.

Health Education Authority (1990) Sugars in the diet. Briefing paper. Health Education Authority, London.

Health Education Authority (1992) *Scientific Basis of Nutrition. A Synopsis of Dietary Reference Values.* Health Education Authority, London.

WHO (1990) Diet, nutrition, and the prevention of chronic diseases. Report of a WHO study group. WHO Technical Report Series 797. WHO, Geneva.

Chapter 3
Healthy Eating

This chapter will consider some practical guidelines which can be used to help individuals to choose a healthy diet. These guidelines are intended for healthy adults who are not overweight. They do not always apply in disease states (see Section 3), although it may just be necessary to change the emphasis of some parts of the diet and stress some points in more detail.

Basic guidelines for healthy eating are to:

- Meet the requirement for essential nutrients
- Look after the vitamins and minerals in the food
- Supply an appropriate amount of energy to maintain ideal body weight
- Choose a diet rich in complex carbohydrates and non-starch polysaccharides (dietary fibre)
- Choose a diet low in fat, particularly saturated fat
- Moderate sugar intake
- Moderate salt intake
- Moderate alcohol intake
- Maintain an adequate fluid intake

Essential nutrients

The most important principle of healthy eating is that the requirement for all essential nutrients should be met. These include protein, essential fatty acids and vitamins and minerals. For further details of functions, food sources and requirements for vitamins and minerals see Appendix 2.

Most foods contain a variety of nutrients but nearly all are deficient in one or more of these and it is therefore essential to eat a variety of foods in moderation. All essential nutrients can be obtained by choosing a mixture of starchy foods such as bread, potatoes, rice or pasta, and plenty of fruit and vegetables, moderate amounts of dairy products, meat, fish, eggs or pulses, and small quantities of spreading fats and cooking oils.

Fruit and vegetables are rich sources of vitamins and minerals but only if they are stored and cooked properly. They should always be stored in a cool dark place and eaten as soon as possible after buying. They should be eaten raw whenever possible or cooked in the minimum amount of water for the shortest possible time. Frozen vegetables should be cooked straight from the freezer. Sodium bicarbonate should never be used when cooking vegetables, and reheating should be avoided. Vegetable water may be used to add to soups and gravy.

Many people continue to be concerned about protein intake because its importance has been emphasised for so long. Protein is a vital nutrient which must be consumed to provide the essential amino acids but by following the dietary advice in this chapter protein intake will take care of itself.

Energy

The appropriate amount of energy to obtain is that which maintains body weight in the ideal range. Body weight should be maintained by careful attention to both energy intake and physical activity. Practical guidelines for controlling body weight are given in Chapter 19.

Estimated average requirements for energy can be found in Appendix 1, but these should always be used with caution because individuals vary so much in their requirements: what is appropriate for one person is not appropriate for another. They vary with age, sex and level of activity, but can also vary between people who are apparently similar in terms of all these factors.

Units

The unit of energy with which most people are familiar is the calorie (cal) and 1000 calories is equivalent to 1 kilocalorie (kcal) or 1 Calorie (Cal). The newer international system of units (SI) measures energy in joules (J). The following formula can be used to convert from one system to the other.

1 kcal = 4.18 kJ
1 MJ = 240 kcal

How energy is obtained

Energy is not itself a nutrient but is obtained from carbohydrate, fat, protein and alcohol in the diet. Carbohydrate and protein both supply about 16.8 kJ (4 kcal)/g while alcohol supplies 29.4 kJ (7 kcal) and fat 37.8 kJ (9 kcal)/g.

Much of the debate about healthy eating has focused on the proportions of energy intake which should be provided by carbohydrate, fat and protein. Current dietary guidelines for intakes of these nutrients are therefore expressed as a proportion of energy intake. This takes account of the fact that different people have different energy requirements.

Both the World Health Organization (WHO) and the Committee on Medical Aspects of Food Policy (COMA) recommend that we should derive about half of our energy from starchy carbohydrates. Thus, if the diet provides 8.4 MJ (1000 kcal)/d, 4.2 MJ (1000 kcal) should come from complex carbohydrates. Carbohydrate supplies 16.8 kJ (4 kcal)/g so this means an intake of 250 g of complex carbohydrates a day.

Although nearly 50% of our energy intake in the UK is derived from carbohydrate, nearly one-third of this carbohydrate comes from sugar.

Complex carbohydrates

Complex carbohydrates are a diverse group of substances which can be classified as starch and non-starch polysaccharides (NSP).

Functions of starchy foods

Starchy foods are filling without being fattening. In the past, people were led to believe that bread, potatoes and cereals were fattening. However, served on their own they are not. It is only when these foods are served or cooked with fat or fatty sauces that they are high in calories. A slice of bread provides about 340 kJ (80 kcal) but when spread with butter it provides about 630 kJ (150 kcal).

Starchy foods are also a good source of essential nutrients including some vitamins, minerals and protein. Reducing the intake of meat, cheese and eggs and increasing the intake of starchy foods is extremely unlikely to prejudice protein intake. In any case most people in Britain eat far more protein than they require. Increasing the intake of starchy foods will also help to reduce fat intake towards recommended levels.

Dietary advice

Complex carbohydrates should provide about half the dietary energy. In practice this means basing the diet on starchy foods. Bread, potatoes, rice or pasta should form the main part of every meal.

Instead of meat with potatoes and a small amount of vegetables people should be encouraged to think in terms of potatoes, rice or pasta with a large serving of vegetables and a small amount of meat, fish, cheese or pulses. The starchy parts of the meal should be planned first and then the meat, fish or cheese. This is quite a change in emphasis for many people in Britain and one that can therefore only be achieved gradually.

As a rough guide, the recommended intake of complex carbohydrates can be achieved by consuming three to four servings a day from the following list of foods:

- Bread of any kind including wholemeal, brown, white, granary, soft grain, 'high fibre' white bread, pitta, chapatti, naan, crispbread, muffins, crumpets, bagels and currant bread
- Breakfast cereals

- Cereals including rice, pasta, oats, barley, rye, cracked wheat (bulghur), couscous, millet, plain popcorn and cornmeal
- Potatoes, sweet potatoes, cassava, green bananas, yams and plantain

Fruit and vegetables

As part of the advice to choose a diet rich in complex carbohydrates, individuals should also be advised to consume plenty of fruit and vegetables. These have always been considered to be part of a healthy diet because they are rich in vitamins and minerals. They are also bulky and low in energy, providing a healthy alternative to fatty and sugary snacks.

Recent research has focused on the importance of the anti-oxidant nutrients, vitamins C and E, beta-carotene, selenium and also folic acid in the prevention of diseases such as coronary heart disease and cancer. Fruit and vegetables – particularly the green and orange varieties – are rich in the anti-oxidant nutrients and folic acid, and current guidelines advise the consumption of five or more servings of fruit and vegetables every day, including one serving of pulses or nuts.

Many people in Britain eat fruit only once or twice a week and a serving of vegetables perhaps every other day. Such advice can therefore mean quite a drastic change, and a gradual increase should be encouraged. Fruit is expensive, and pharmacists should be particularly sensitive in their advice to people on low incomes (see Chapter 24) who may find it difficult to achieve this target.

As a rough guide the recommended change could be achieved by consuming a glass of fruit juice, two pieces of fresh fruit or two servings of tinned or stewed fruit and one serving of green vegetables or a salad every day. In addition, pulses should be consumed about three times a week. This could be a small can of baked beans, a serving of kidney beans in a casserole or salad, or a serving of lentil soup.

Non-starch polysaccharides (NSP)

Composition

NSP is now the preferred scientific term for dietary fibre. This is very confusing for the general public who have only recently got used to the term 'fibre' after many years' usage of the term 'roughage'. The reason for the change is that 'fibre' is not a very precise term and it cannot be measured accurately in the laboratory. Consequently, this has led to a great deal of disagreement as to the amount of fibre in various foods. NSP can, however, be measured with reasonable accuracy, and it is the major component of dietary fibre.

Practically, this means that foods which are high in NSP are also high in dietary fibre. Until the term NSP is more widely known by the general public, pharmacists should continue to use 'fibre' or even 'roughage' if these words are better understood, and be prepared to explain the newer terminology if asked about it.

NSP is not quantitatively the same as dietary fibre. For example, 12 g of NSP is roughly equivalent to 20 g of dietary fibre. This will have implications for food labelling in the future as NSP comes into more common usage. If people are interested in studying food labels at this level of detail, they may believe that their favourite breakfast cereal has less 'fibre' than they thought it had. For example, a breakfast cereal may contain 17 g of dietary fibre and 13 g of NSP/100 g.

There are two types of NSP, soluble and insoluble, and they vary in their physiological effects.

Functions

In the small intestine the overall effect of NSP is to slow down and regulate the digestive process. For example NSP reduces the rate of glucose absorption. This has important implications for diabetic patients in controlling blood glucose and insulin levels (see Chapter 6).

NSP appears to have an effect on cholesterol metabolism by altering the rate of recycling of bile. Soluble NSP has a greater influence than insoluble NSP and may help to lower blood cholesterol.

In the large intestine, NSP adds bulk to the faeces and thus helps to prevent constipation. In this respect, insoluble NSP is more important than soluble NSP.

Dietary advice

Current dietary guidelines recommend that the average intake of NSP for the population should be about 18 g of NSP a day. This is roughly equivalent to 30 g of dietary fibre. Figures from The National Food Survey (1999) show that current intake is about 12 g a day. This has changed little in the past five years. Wholegrain breads, cereals and pulses are the richest sources of NSP, with fruits and vegetables supplying more modest amounts. The richest sources of soluble NSP include pulses, oats, rye and barley whereas insoluble NSP is found principally in wheat, rice and some vegetables. The dietary fibre and NSP content of some commonly eaten foods are shown in Table 3.1.

Some practical suggestions for increasing NSP intake include:

- choosing wholemeal bread. Pitta bread and muffins are also made in wholemeal varieties
- choosing a wholegrain breakfast cereal
- choosing wholemeal pasta and brown rice
- eating more potatoes, particularly with the skin
- using wholemeal flour for baking or half wholemeal and half white flour
- eating pulses such as dried beans and lentils three times a week
- eating plenty of fruit and vegetables

Table 3.1   Approximate fibre and NSP content of various foods (g/portion).

Food and portion	Total fibre	[NSP]
Bread		
Brown, 2 slices	4	2.5
Brown roll, 1	3.5	2
Chapattis, 1	5	–
Croissant, 1	1.5	1
French stick, 2 small slices	4	1
Granary, 2 slices	4	2.5
Naan bread, 1	4	3
Poppadoms, 2	2	–
White, 2 slices	3	1.5
White roll, 1	2	1
Wholemeal, 2 slices	5	4
Wholemeal roll, 1	5	4
Breakfast cereals		
All-Bran, 1 bowl (50 g)	15	12
Bran Flakes, 1 bowl (40 g)	8	6
Corn Flakes, 1 bowl (30 g)	1	0.5
Mucsli, 1 bowl (90 g)	8	6
Porridge, 1 bowl (160 g)	1.5	1.5
Rice Krispies, 1 bowl (30 g)	0.5	0.5
Shredded Wheat, 2 pieces (40 g)	4.5	4
Special K, 1 bowl (30 g)	1	1
Sugar Puffs, 1 bowl (50 g)	2.5	2
Weetabix, 2 pieces (40 g)	3.5	3
Weetaflakes, 1 bowl (40 g)	5	4
Pasta and rice – cooked		
Pasta, wholemeal, 1 serving (150 g)	6	4
white, 1 serving (150 g)	3	2.5
Rice, brown, 1 serving (150 g)	2.5	1.5
white 1 serving (150 g)	1	0.5
Pulses – cooked		
Baked beans, 1 200 g can	13	6.5
Dhal, chickpea, 1 serving (150 g)	8	–
lentil, 1 serving (150 g)	3	–
Hummus, 1 serving (60 g)	2	1.5
Kidney beans, 1 serving (100 g)	7	5
Lentil soup, 1 bowl	4	2
Nuts		
Mixed nuts (25 g)	2	1.5
Peanuts, 1 small packet (25 g)	2	1.5
Peanut butter, in 1 sandwich	0.5	0.5
Vegetables		
Broccoli, 1 serving (90 g)	3	2.5
Brussels sprouts, 1 serving (100 g)	3	3.5
Cabbage 1 serving (70 g)	2	1.5
Carrots, 1 serving (70 g)	2	2
Runner beans, 1 serving (105 g)	3	2

Cont.

Table 3.1 Cont.

Food and portion	Total fibre	[NSP]
Peas, frozen, 1 serving (70 g)	6	4
Plantain, 1 serving (80 g)	2	1.5
Potatoes, boiled, 1 serving (150 g)	1.5	1.5
baked, 1 jacket (150 g)	3	2.5
sweet, 1 serving (150 g)	3	3
Sweetcorn, 1 serving (70 g)	3.5	2.5
Tomatoes, 2	1.5	1.0
Yams, 1 serving (130 g)	5	2.5
Fruit		
Apple, 1 eating	2	1.5
Apricots, dried, 4	6	5
Bananas, 1	1.5	1.0
Blackberries, 15	5	2.5
Orange, 1	3	3
Plums, 3	2	1.5

It is important to eat a diet containing NSP-rich foods, but the most important advice is to increase the consumption of starchy carbohydrates. Foods rich in NSP are normally rich in starch too, but foods rich in starch are not necessarily good sources of NSP. White bread, for example, contains less NSP than wholemeal but just as much starch. If individuals dislike wholemeal bread, it is far better for them to continue eating white bread than to eat no bread at all. In other words, white bread is good, but wholemeal is better still.

Fat

Composition

Most of the fat in the diet is in the form of triglycerides which are composed of one molecule of glycerol and three molecules of fatty acids. (The characteristics of dietary fat are determined largely by the nature of the fatty acids. Fatty acids may be saturated, monounsaturated or polyunsaturated depending on the number of double bonds in the molecule.)

Saturated fatty acids

Saturated fatty acids contain no double bonds and are solid at room temperature. They are not essential components of the diet and may be harmful in large quantities. The main sources of saturated fatty acids in the diet are butter and dairy products and foods containing them, coconut oil and the fat on meat.

Monounsaturated fatty acids

Monounsaturated fatty acids are liquid at room temperatures and contain one double bond. The main dietary source is olive oil; peanut oil (groundnut oil) is also a good source.

Polyunsaturated fatty acids

Polyunsaturated fatty acids contain two or more double bonds and they may be liquid or semi-solid at room temperature. Unlike the saturated and monounsaturated fatty acids, polyunsaturated fatty acids – at least the parent polyunsaturates – cannot be synthesised in the body and they must be obtained from the diet. Hence they are known as the essential fatty acids.

There are two types of essential fatty acids, the n-6 family and the n-3 family. The main n-6 fatty acid in the diet is linoleic acid, which is found in vegetable oils such as safflower oil and sunflower oil, nuts and lean meat. Alpha-linolenic acid is the main n-3 fatty acid and is found in some vegetable oils, particularly soya bean oil.

Both linoleic and alpha-linolenic acid are metabolised in the body to form longer chain and more unsaturated fatty acids (see Fig. 3.1). Two of the longer chain derivatives of the n-3 series, eicosapentaenoic acid and doc-

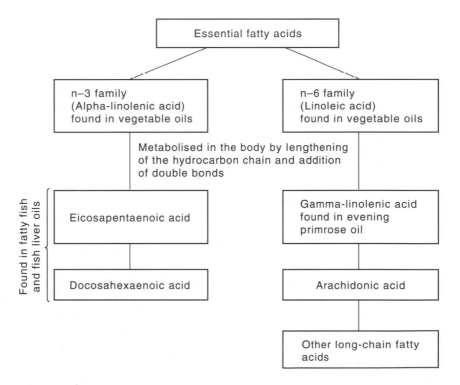

Fig. 3.1   Metabolism of essential fatty acids.

osahexaenoic acid, are also found in fatty fish such as tuna, sardines, herring and mackerel. Dietary supplements of fish oils and fish liver oils are also good sources.

Trans fatty acids

The double bonds in all naturally occurring fatty acids have a *cis* configuration but can be isomerised to the *trans* form during the partial hydrogenation of oils and fats by the food industry. *Trans* fatty acids appear to have similar biological effects to saturated fatty acids.

Function of fats

Dietary fats have a number of important functions. They serve as a source of the essential fatty acids, and some fat is required for the absorption of the fat-soluble vitamins. Fat is a concentrated source of energy and it usually improves the palatability of food.

Recommendations

Although fat is an important part of the diet, many people eat far more than is necessary. Dietary guidelines suggest that no more than 33% of energy should come from total fat and no more than 10% from saturated fat. In a diet providing about 8.4 MJ (2000 kcal)/d this means an upper limit of about 75 g of total fat and 22 g of saturated fat. Although total fat intake is declining in the UK, it still represents about 38% of energy intake. Saturated fat represents about 14% of energy intake, so there is still some way to go to reach the recommendations.

The amount of fat obtained from different foods in the British diet is shown in Fig. 3.2.

Reducing fat intake

The most important advice to give about dietary fat is to reduce the total amount consumed. Arguments about which type of fat to use, e.g. butter or margarine, are likely to continue. Whatever fats are chosen they should be used sparingly.

The most positive way to achieve a reduction in fat intake is to recommend an increase in the intake of complex carbohydrates, i.e. to base meals on bread, cereals, potatoes, pasta or rice. By having larger servings of these foods the fat content of the diet is likely to fall because individuals may be too full or will not have enough room on their plates for large amounts of foods high in fat. For example, four thin slices of bread a day can be replaced with two thick slices. Without even a mention of fat intake, the quantity of butter or spread used should decrease by half.

It is also important to consider the fat content of foods. On food labels fat content is normally expressed in terms of weight, i.e. as grams of fat per 100 g

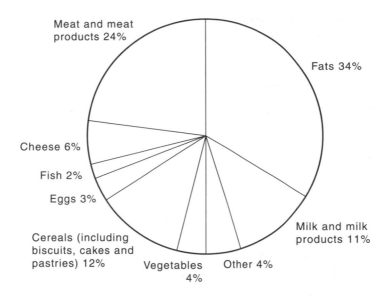

Fig. 3.2   Percentage of fat obtained from foods in the British diet.

of food. However, dietary guidelines make recommendations in terms of percentage of total energy.

Fat content shown as a percentage by weight is usually much lower than fat content expressed as a proportion of energy (see Table 3.2). Foods labelled as containing 5 or 10% fat are not necessarily low in fat, and food labels may eventually describe fat content in terms of percentage energy. Any food in which fat provides more than 33% of the total energy cannot be considered to be low in fat.

The fat content of food is not always a good indicator of the food's contribution to daily fat consumption. The serving size and frequency of consumption must always be taken into account. Double cream, for example, is high in fat but if only consumed once a month it makes very little difference to overall fat consumption. Full fat milk, on the other hand, may be consumed in large quantities every day, and although it is lower in fat than double cream it makes a much greater contribution to daily fat intake. Replacement of full fat milk by skimmed or semi-skimmed milk is likely to have a much greater effect on fat consumption than avoiding cream completely.

Margarines, spreads and oils

Margarines, spreads and oils are a significant source of fat in the diet and there is a great deal of confusion about their fat content (see Fig. 3.3). Margarine, including polyunsaturated margarine, is no lower in fat than butter, and vegetable oils high in polyunsaturates are no lower in fat than lard and dripping (see Fig. 3.4).

Table 3.2 Fat content of various foods.

Food	Fat % by weight	Fat % energy
Milk, cream and yoghurt		
Whole milk	4	55
Semi-skimmed milk	1.5	29
Skimmed milk	0.1	3
Double cream	48	96
Single cream	19	86
Whipping cream	39	94
Whole milk yoghurt (plain)	3	34
Whole milk yoghurt (fruit)	3	26
Low fat yoghurt (plain)	0.8	13
Low fat yoghurt (fruit)	0.7	7
Greek yoghurt	9	70
Butter, spreads and oil		
Butter	82	100
Margarine	82	100
Polyunsaturated margarine	82	100
Low fat spread	40	92
Very low fat spread	25	82
5% fat spread	5	45
Cheese		
Blue cheese	30	78
Brie	27	76
Camembert	24	73
Cottage cheese	4	37
Cottage cheese (low fat)	1.5	17
Cream cheese	48	98
Edam	25	67
Feta	20	72
Fromage frais	7	56
Fromage frais (low fat)	0.2	3
Hard cheese, e.g. Cheddar, Leicester	34	74
Low fat hard cheese	15	52
White cheese, e.g. Cheshire	31	74
Meat and meat products		
Bacon (grilled)	34	76
Beefburgers (grilled)	17	58
Chicken (no skin, roast)	5	30
Chicken (with skin, roast)	14	58
Lamb chop (fat removed, grilled)	7	52
Leg of lamb (lean, roast)	8	48
Lamb's liver (fried)	14	54
Mince (stewed)	15	59
Pork chop (fat removed, grilled)	6	40
Pork chop (with fat, grilled)	19	66
Pork pie	27	65
Pork sausage (grilled)	25	71
Pork sausage (low fat, grilled)	14	55

Cont.

Table 3.2   Cont.

Food	Fat % by weight	Fat % energy
Rump steak (fat removed, grilled)	6	32
Sausage roll	36	68
Sirloin (lean, roast)	9	45
Steak (stewed)	11	44
Topside (lean, roast)	4	23
Turkey (no skin, roast)	3	19
Turkey (with skin, roast)	6	32
Fish		
Kipper (baked)	11	49
Mackerel (fried)	11	53
Mackerel (smoked)	30	77
Sardines (canned, drained)	14	58
Tuna (canned in oil, drained)	9	43
Tuna (canned in brine, drained)	0.6	5
White fish (e.g. cod, haddock, plaice, grilled or baked)	1	10
White fish fried in batter	10	45
White fish fried in breadcrumbs	8	41
Chips and crisps		
Chips (chip shop)	12	45
French fries	16	51
Oven chips	4	22
Crisps	38	63
Crisps (low fat)	22	41
Biscuits, cakes and chocolate		
Cream crackers	16	33
Digestive biscuits, chocolate	24	44
plain	21	40
Sandwich biscuits (e.g. custard creams)	26	46
Tea biscuits	17	33
Chocolate eclair	20	60
Croissants	20	50
Doughnuts	20	45
Fruit cake	13	33
Sponge cake	26	51
Chocolate	30	51

Using a margarine or cooking oil rich in polyunsaturates or mono-unsaturates will help to reduce the intake of saturated fat but not that of total fat. For individuals of normal weight a polyunsaturated margarine is a healthy choice, but for individuals who are overweight it is better to choose a low or very low fat spread because this will help to reduce their energy intake. Butter need not be avoided; it should be reserved to add occasionally to those foods where the taste of butter is considered to be particularly important.

Unless specific advice about fats has been given by a dietitian, it is probably

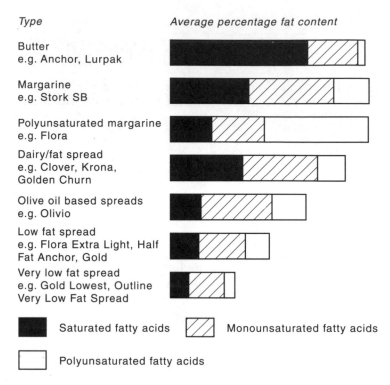

Fig. 3.3 Fat content of butter, margarine and spreads (these data should be used as a guide only; figures may change).

wise to advise the use of a mixture of types of spreads, oils and fats and to reduce the quantity of whichever is used.

Low fat foods

There are now several 'low' and 'reduced' fat alternatives, including milks, yoghurts, cheeses, spreads, sausages, beefburgers, salad dressings, mayonnaise, crisps and chips. 'Low fat' or 'reduced fat' normally means that the product contains less fat than the ordinary equivalent but not necessarily that the food is low in fat (see Table 3.2). Food labels need to be studied carefully.

Skimmed and semi-skimmed milks and low fat yoghurts are genuinely low in fat but low fat spreads are not. Low fat spreads contain 40 times as much fat as low fat yoghurt, and low fat sausages and reduced fat hard cheese contain ten times as much fat as reduced fat cottage cheese. 'Low' or 'reduced' fat is a comparative term, not an absolute one. Misunderstanding of these terms may encourage people to make liberal use of these products with the result that fat intake is not reduced. However, if any low fat product is used to replace a full fat variety on a weight for weight basis, fat intake will fall.

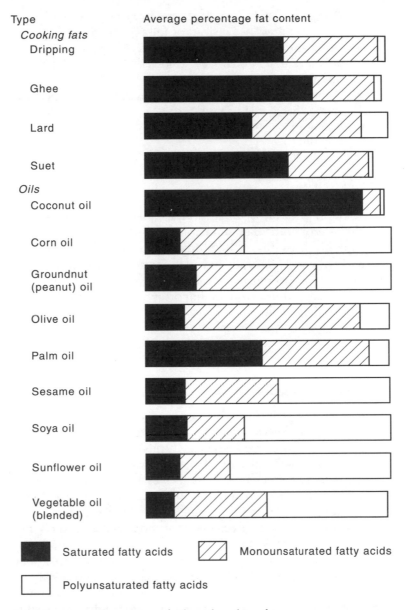

Fig. 3.4   Percentage fat content of oils and cooking fats.

Some practical suggestions which will help to reduce fat intake include:

- Choosing skimmed or semi-skimmed milk rather than whole milk
- Grilling, microwaving, baking, steaming or boiling foods rather than frying
- Choosing chicken (without the skin), fish and lean meat rather than fatty meat; trimming all fat from meat

- Using low fat cheeses, yoghurts, fromage frais and low fat mayonnaises and salad dressings instead of full fat varieties
- Using as little fat or oil as possible in cooking; it is better to use oils rich in polyunsaturates, such as sunflower or soya oil, or those rich in mono-unsaturates, such as olive oil, rather than lard or dripping
- Using as little spread on bread as possible; moist sandwich fillings such as cream cheese and peanut butter can be eaten without spread
- Eating foods such as pastries, pies, biscuits, cakes and crisps only occasionally

Cholesterol

Some fat in the diet is in the form of cholesterol. Many people are confused by cholesterol in the diet and cholesterol in the blood. Manufacturers tend to exploit this confusion by producing low cholesterol foods. Dietary cholesterol, however, generally has an insignificant effect on serum cholesterol. The majority of people do not need to worry about cholesterol in the diet. Saturated fat is much more important. Cholesterol is found mainly in eggs, liver and shellfish.

Sugar

Composition and function

Dietary sugars include the monosaccharides glucose and fructose and the disaccharides sucrose, lactose and maltose. Sugars are present in the diet in two forms. These are known as intrinsic sugar and extrinsic sugar. Intrinsic sugar is an integral part of the cell wall of foods (inside the cell) and is therefore found in whole fruits such as apples and oranges. Extrinsic sugar is sugar that has been removed from the cell wall (outside the cell) and is found in fruit juice, honey, syrup, molasses and table sugar.

The distinction between extrinsic and intrinsic sugars is important because they are metabolised in different ways. Sugar which is part of the cell wall of fruits is absorbed relatively slowly and produces a more gradual rise in blood glucose and insulin levels. Extrinsic sugars, on the other hand, are absorbed much faster and result in rapid rises in blood glucose and insulin levels. This has implications in the dietary management of diabetes mellitus (see Chapter 6).

Many people believe that sugar and foods containing it 'give them energy'. Sugar does provide energy, but a couple of boiled sweets provide no more energy than an apple. The energetic feeling resulting from sugar consumption is a consequence of the rapid rise in blood glucose, but this falls just as quickly because of the rapid increase in insulin levels. The need for a further sugary snack returns quite quickly.

Foods containing extrinsic sugar tend to be consumed much more rapidly than foods containing intrinsic sugar. For example, it takes far less time to drink a glass of apple juice than it does to eat an apple. Extrinsic sugar (usually sucrose) is often combined with fat in foods which are highly palatable (e.g. chocolate). Both these factors, together with the fact that extrinsic sugar tends to produce rapid rises and falls in blood glucose, may encourage excessive energy intake.

Dietary advice

Dietary guidelines recommend that no more than 10% of energy intake should be obtained from extrinsic sugar. This figure excludes the lactose in milk which is also extrinsic but which is considered to be a special case. This means that for a diet providing 8.4 MJ (2000 kcal) the upper limit for extrinsic sugar intake is 50 g.

Alternative forms of sugar (e.g. brown sugar, raw cane sugar, syrup, molasses, glucose syrup and honey) are often believed to be beneficial, but there is nothing to be gained by substituting any of these for white sugar.

Individuals may need guidance on which foods are high in sugar (see Table 3.3). Apart from the most obvious sources such as sweets, cakes, jams and chocolate, sugar is also found in substantial amounts in breakfast cereals, fizzy drinks and even in savoury foods such as pickles, chutneys, ketchups and baked beans.

Table 3.3 Sugar content of various foods (g/portion).

Food and portion	Sugar
Sweet spreads and sugar	
Honey, on 1 slice of bread	8
Jam, on 1 slice of bread	7
reduced sugar	3
Marmalade, on 1 slice of bread	7
Sugar (brown or white), 1 teaspoon	5
Sweets and chocolates	
Boiled sweets (4 oz; 112 g)	87
Fruit gums, 1 tube	15
Fruit pastilles, 1 tube	25
Mars bar, 1	43
Toffees (4 oz; 112 g)	70
Cakes and biscuits	
Chocolate eclair, 1	3
Digestive biscuits, chocolate, 2	10
plain, 2	5
Doughnut, jam, 1	10
Fruit cake, 1 slice	25
Sandwich biscuits (e.g. custard creams), 2	7
Sponge cake, 1 slice	15
Tea biscuits, 2	3

Cont.

Table 3.3   Cont.

Food and portion	Sugar
Drinks	
Coke, 1 can	30
Lemonade, 1 glass	11
Lucozade, 1 glass	17
Orange juice, unsweetened, 1 glass	17
Orange squash, 1 glass	14
Ribena, 1 glass	30
Pickles and soups	
Chutney, 1 serving	15
Sweet pickle, 1 serving	10
Tomato ketchup, 1 serving	5
Tomato soup, canned, 1 bowl	5
low calorie, 1 bowl	4
Breakfast cereals	
All-Bran, 1 bowl	10
Bran Flakes, 1 bowl	8
Corn Flakes, 1 bowl	2
Frosties, 1 bowl	20
Muesli, 1 bowl	26
no added sugar	16
Rice Crispies, 1 bowl	4
Shredded Wheat, 2 pieces	0.3
Special K, 1 bowl	5
Sugar Puffs, 1 bowl	28
Weetabix, 2 pieces	2
Weetaflakes, 1 bowl	8
Miscellaneous	
Baked beans, 200 g can	12
reduced sugar	6
Peaches, canned in syrup, 6 halves	16
canned in juice, 6 halves	10

Claims about sugar on food labels can be confusing. 'Reduced sugar' means that the product contains less sugar than the ordinary equivalent but not necessarily that the food is low in sugar. 'Sugar-free' means that a product is free from sucrose but not necessarily free from other extrinsic sugars; a 'sugar-free' product may be sweetened with concentrated fruit juice or honey. 'No added sugar' means that sugar is not added in any form, but unsweetened products such as fruit juice are rich in free sugars. Food labels should be checked for ingredients such as glucose, dextrose, corn syrup, glucose syrup, syrup, molasses, honey, treacle and concentrated fruit juice which all mean sugar.

Some practical suggestions which will help to moderate sugar intake include:

- Avoiding sugar in tea and coffee or adding an artificial sweetener
- Choosing low calorie or 'diet' drinks rather than sugary squashes or fizzy drinks
- Diluting unsweetened fruit juices with water
- Choosing breakfast cereals which are not coated in sugar or honey and avoiding extra sugar
- Using honey or jam sparingly
- Reducing the amount of sugar used in recipes
- Choosing tinned fruit in natural juice or water instead of syrup
- Replacing sweets, biscuits, chocolates and cakes as much as possible with fruit

Salt

Sodium is an essential part of the diet but most people consume far more than they need and there is potential benefit in reducing current intake. A low sodium diet maybe prescribed in hypertension (see Chapter 5), renal failure (see Chapter 11) and liver failure (see Chapter 12), but initial dietary advice for such patients must be given by a dietitian.

Salt is added both in cooking and at the table and could be reduced or avoided in both these situations. Salt is available in various forms including iodised salt and sea salt; these do not have a different sodium content from ordinary salt.

Salt substitutes containing potassium are available and may be used to reduce sodium intake but they should be avoided by patients with renal failure and by those taking angiotensin-converting enzyme (ACE) inhibitors, potassium-sparing diuretics and cyclosporin.

A substantial proportion of sodium intake comes from processed foods, particularly smoked and canned meats and fish and also breakfast cereals (see Table 3.4). Food labels should be checked for the words 'brine' and 'smoked' and also for ingredients such as monosodium glutamate (MSG), sodium bicarbonate, sodium sulphate, sodium chloride and sodium nitrite.

Some practical suggestions which will help to moderate salt intake include:

- Avoiding or reducing the amount of salt in cooking
- Avoiding adding salt at the table
- Choosing processed food labelled 'low in salt' or 'no added salt'
- Restricting the frequency of consumption of 'high' salt food to twice or three times a week
- Replacing salty snacks with unsalted nuts, fruit or plain popcorn.

Alcohol

Alcohol is not an essential part of the diet but it has important social functions and, in moderation, it may have some beneficial influence in the

Table 3.4   Salt content of various foods.

High sodium (250 mg or more in a serving)
Meat and meat products
   Bacon, black pudding, corned beef, ham, luncheon meat, meat pies, pâté,
   salami, salt beef, sausages, tongue
 	
Fish
   Canned fish, shellfish, smoked fish
 	
Cereals, biscuits, snacks
   Most breakfast cereals
   Bread
   Biscuits, crispbreads
   Potato crisps, salted nuts
 	
Pickles and soups
   Ketchup, mayonnaise, pickles, salad cream, sauces, Bovril, Oxo, Marmite,
   baking powder
   Canned and packet soups
 	
Vegetables
   Canned vegetables including baked beans (and reduced salt baked beans)
 	
Cheese
   Most cheeses, particularly blue cheeses and Edam
 	
Medium sodium (25–250 mg in a serving)
Milk, butter, margarine
Some mineral waters, e.g. Buxton, Strathmore, Vichy
 	
Low sodium (25 mg or less in a serving)
Fresh and frozen vegetables and fruit
Fresh and frozen meat, poultry and fish
Rice and most pasta
Some breakfast cereals, e.g. Shredded Wheat and home-made muesli
Unsalted products, e.g. butter, margarine
Unsalted nuts
Some mineral waters, e.g. Evian, Highland Spring, Perrier, Spa, Volvic, Vittel

prevention of coronary heart disease. However, it is a fairly concentrated source of energy (29.4 MJ or 7 kcal/g), and consumption should be taken into account in any individual who needs to lose weight.

Alcohol should not be consumed during pregnancy and care should be taken when driving, particularly if sedative drugs are being taken at the same time (see Chapter 26). Moderation in alcohol intake is particularly important for patients with hypertension (see Chapter 5), diabetes mellitus (see Chapter 6), peptic ulcer (see Chapter 8) and gout (see Chapter 13).

Safe limits

Alcohol is measured in units. Recommended safe limits are considered to be for a woman 2–3 units a day and for a man 3–4 units a day. These guidelines have replaced the older weekly limits which, it was considered, did nothing to discourage 'binge' drinking on a Saturday night. It should be noted that these are safe limits and not definite recommendations.

There is confusion amongst both health professionals and the general public about the system of alcohol units, and pharmacists should be able to give a clear explanation when giving advice about alcohol. As a rough guide, one unit of alcohol can be found in each of the following drinks:

- Half a pint of ordinary beer or lager
- A quarter of a pint of strong beer or lager
- A third of a pint of ordinary strength cider
- A quarter of a pint of strong cider
- One single bar measure of whisky, gin or brandy
- One glass of table wine
- One bar measure of sherry, vermouth or port
- One bar measure of liqueurs

There is a wide variation in the alcohol content of different brands of the same type of drink. Home measures tend to be larger than bar measures. Measures of spirits tend to be greater in Northern Ireland and some parts of Scotland than in England.

There are a number of 'low alcohol' and 'alcohol-free' drinks on the market, including lagers, ciders and wine, but the labelling of these drinks is frequently confusing. Alcohol-free drinks are not totally devoid of alcohol but usually contain less than 0.05%. Low alcohol drinks usually contain between 0.05 and 1.2% alcohol but labels should be studied carefully.

Fluid

Requirement

Water constitutes about 70% of the total body weight and it is the medium in which almost all metabolic processes take place. A constant supply of water is therefore essential and an average adult living in a temperate climate requires about 2500 ml a day. Water is a constituent of all drinks and most foods, especially fruit and vegetables, but it is also found in solid foods such as bread, meat and fish.

Drinks

Most of the water requirement is supplied by drinks. Non-alcoholic drinks include tea, coffee, milk, water and soft drinks.

Tea and coffee

There is a great variety of tea and coffee and some teas have added flavours such as lemon or bergamot. Herbal teas are steadily increasing in popularity and are often drunk in the belief that they are healthier than ordinary tea because they are claimed not to contain caffeine or tannins. However, some herbal teas (e.g. raspberry) stimulate the uterus and, if drunk in large quantities during pregnancy, may induce abortion. Chamomile tea causes hypersensitivity reactions in susceptible people and comfrey contains potentially toxic substances. Herb teas are therefore best used in small amounts as part of a varied diet.

Tea and coffee do not provide significant amounts of energy unless milk and/or sugar are added but they do contain caffeine. Caffeine is a mild stimulant which increases the heart rate and urine production. Consumption of coffee and tea should be restricted to no more than five cups a day. Coffee and tea are also available in decaffeinated forms.

Soft drinks

There is a great deal of confusion about fruit juices, fruit drinks and fruit cordials. Some contain added sugar and some do not, so labels should be studied carefully. Even unsweetened fruit juices contain large amounts of extrinsic sugar so are better diluted with water.

Soft, fizzy drinks have an average sugar content of 10% but 'diet' drinks, either devoid of sugar or containing reduced amounts, are available. Cola drinks normally contain caffeine but they are also available in decaffeinated forms.

Tap water

Tap water is generally safe to drink in the UK; it is monitored for safety and must meet certain standards. Fluoride levels vary in different areas and details can be obtained from the local Water Company. Nitrate levels may exceed limits set by the EU in some parts of the UK such as East Anglia but the levels are below those known to cause harmful effects.

In chalk or limestone areas the water will be hard and contain considerable quantities of calcium and magnesium. In a granite area the water is softer and is lower in mineral content than hard water. Consumption of hard water may reduce the risk of coronary heart disease.

Several devices are available which soften and filter tap water. Some work on the principle of ion exchange which replaces the calcium and magnesium in the water with sodium. These should not be used by people on low sodium diets or to make up infant feeds. More modern water softeners replace the calcium and magnesium with hydrogen ions and the sodium content is not increased.

Mineral water

Mineral and spa waters have been used for centuries but nutritionally they offer no advantage over tap water. Nevertheless they often taste better, and consumption has increased markedly in recent years. They are a useful alternative to soft drinks and alcohol. Some mineral waters are carbonated and some are still; some are 'natural' while others are manufactured. The main difference between these varieties is one of taste. They all contain mineral salts, including sodium, potassium, magnesium and calcium, but the levels vary across the brands. Low and medium sodium mineral waters are listed in Table 3.4.

Conclusion

The box below summarises some general guidelines for healthy eating. Pharmacists should not attempt to communicate more than two or three of these points at once, not only because people will have difficulty in remembering so much information, but also because dietary changes are difficult to make and should be attempted gradually.

General guidelines for healthy eating.

(1) Base all meals on starchy foods, such as bread, cereals, pasta, rice or potatoes

(2) Emphasise starchy foods which are high in NSP

(3) Eat five servings of fruit and vegetables each day

(4) Eat pulses such as lentils, chickpeas and beans two or three times a week

(5) Choose skimmed or semi-skimmed milk rather than whole milk

(6) Choose low fat cheeses and yoghurts

(7) Choose lean meat

(8) Eat poultry without the skin

(9) Increase fish intake, including fatty fish such as mackerel, herring, tuna and sardines

(10) Use butter, spreads and cooking oils sparingly

(11) Grill, microwave or bake rather than fry

(12) Use sugar sparingly

(13) Reserve chocolate, sweets, cakes, biscuits and crisps for occasional use only

(14) Use salt and high-salt foods sparingly

(15) Keep within the recommended limits when drinking alcohol

(16) Drink plenty of fluid

These guidelines have now been translated into what is considered to be a more understandable and useful format for the general public. This is in the form of a National Food Guide, The Balance of Good Health, which was developed by the Ministry of Agriculture, Fisheries and Food, and the Health Education Authority. This is shown as a tilted plate (Fig. 3.5) with divisions of various sizes, each representing one of five food groups to illustrate the types and properties of foods needed to achieve a healthy, well balanced diet.

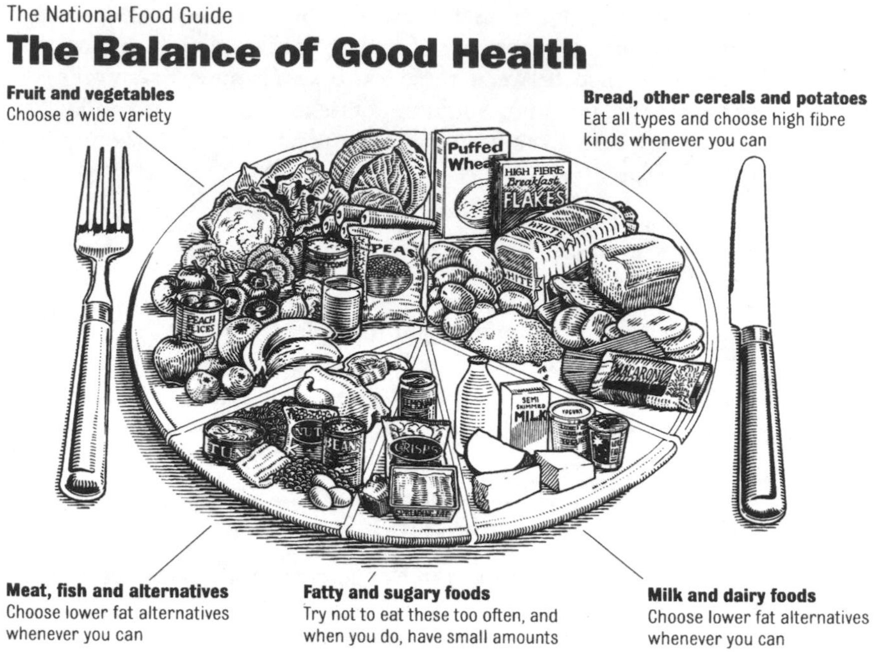

The National Food Guide

The Balance of Good Health

Fruit and vegetables
Choose a wide variety

Bread, other cereals and potatoes
Eat all types and choose high fibre
kinds whenever you can

Meat, fish and alternatives
Choose lower fat alternatives
whenever you can

Fatty and sugary foods
Try not to eat these too often, and
when you do, have small amounts

Milk and dairy foods
Choose lower fat alternatives
whenever you can

Fig. 3.5 The National Food Guide. Reproduced by kind permission of the Health Education Authority.

The actual amount of foods consumed will vary between individuals but the properties remain the same. It emphasises the importance of eating a diet with plenty of bread, cereals and potatoes, and fruit and vegetables, and choosing moderate amounts of low-fat meat and dairy produce, with fatty and sugary foods forming a small part of the diet.

Further reading

Health Education Authority (1992) Starch and dietary fibre. A briefing paper. Health Education Authority, London.

Holland, B., Welch, A.A., Unwin, I.D., Buss, D.H., Paul, A.A. and Southgate, D.A.T. (1991) *McCance and Widdowson's The Composition of Foods*, 5th Edition. The Royal Society of Chemistry and the Ministry of Agriculture, Fisheries and Food, London.

Useful leaflets

'Eight guidelines for a healthy diet' available free of charge from Food Sense, London SE99 7TT.

'Enjoy healthy eating' available free of charge from the Distribution Department, Health Education Authority, Trevelyan House, 30 Great Peter Street, London SW1P 2HW.

Useful addresses

Al-Anon Family Groups UK & Eire, 61 Great Dover Street, London SE1 4YF. Tel: 0207 403 0888.

Alcohol Concern, Waterbridge House, 32–36 Loman Street, London SE1 0EE. Tel: 0207 928 7377.

Alcoholics Anonymous (AA), General Service Office, PO Box 1, Stonebow House, Stonebow, York YO1 2NJ. Tel: 01904 644026/7/8/9.

British Dietetic Association, 7th floor, Elizabeth House, 22 Suffolk Street, Queensway, Birmingham B1 1LS. Tel: 0121 643 5483.

British Nutrition Foundation, High Holborn House, 52–54 High Holborn, London WC1V 6RQ. Tel: 0207 404 6504.

Health Education Authority, Trevelyan House, 30 Great Peter Street, London SW1P 2HW. Tel: 0207 222 5300.

National Dairy Council, John Princes Street, London W1M 0AP. Tel: 0207 499 7822.

Chapter 4
Food Safety

Concern about food safety has grown in recent years and this includes fears about food poisoning, additives and agricultural contaminants. Food safety in Britain is controlled in agricultural and farming practice, the food industry, and through the chain to the point of sale. Consumers also have a responsibility for food safety and may require advice on safe food handling practice.

Food poisoning

Food poisoning is an acute illness, usually of microbiological origin, caused by the recent consumption of food or drink. It can also be caused by toxins which are naturally present in the food.

Food poisoning is a widespread problem, and the public are becoming increasingly aware of it. Consequently there has been a growth in the number of reported cases. About 53 000 cases were notified in 1998, but this figure is likely to be a conservative estimate because many cases are not notified. Food poisoning is more common in the summer although it can occur throughout the year.

During the mid 1990s, there was concern about bovine spongiform encephalopathy (BSE), the so-called 'mad cow disease' and the possibility that it could be transmitted to humans. The infective agent responsible for BSE was acquired through incorporation of animal products into cattle feed, and it was the consumption of tissue from bovine brain and spinal cord, used in products such as beefburgers, meat pies and sausages, which was considered to pose the greatest risk to humans. At the end of 1989, the British government stated that British beef products should not contain any brain, spinal cord or lymphoid tissue, but there still exists the possibility that individuals who consumed large quantities of beef products prior to 1989 could be at risk. More research is required to assess the risk to humans and to develop methods of early detection in humans before the onset of clinical symptoms.

Genetically modified (GM) food has also become an area of concern. Genetic modification allows for more rapid breeding of plants to select desired characteristics (eg resistance to pesticides and frost) than traditional methods and therefore offers advantages, especially in farming and food production. No GM crops are yet grown commercially for food in the UK, although several trials are underway. GM foods available in the UK are made mainly from crops grown in the US and include tomato purée, soya, maize, cheese and an array of enzymes used to make a large variety of products such as fizzy drinks, baked goods and dairy produce. There is no evidence that GM foods on sale at the moment pose any risk to human health, although there is not enough evidence yet to state categorically that all GM foods are 100% safe.

Microbiological food poisoning

The most common food poisoning organisms and associated symptoms are shown in Table 4.1.

The most common symptoms of food poisoning are gastrointestinal and often involve diarrhoea and abdominal pain. Pharmacists are often asked for advice about such symptoms and should always bear in mind the possibility of food poisoning.

Susceptible groups of people

Everyone is at risk from food poisoning but certain groups of the population are more vulnerable than others. These groups include:

- Pregnant women and unborn children
- Infants and children (particularly those under 2 years)
- The elderly
- Those who are taking drugs with an immunosuppressant action, e.g. azathioprine and drugs used for treating cancer
- Those who are immunocompromised because of illness such as AIDS, or alcoholics, drug abusers and transplant patients

Causes

Food can be contaminated by bacteria at any stage from production to consumption. The government, the European Union and local Environmental Health Officers impose a series of tests which start with the farmer and continue right through the food chain including the manufacturer, distributor and retailer.

The consumer is the last person to handle the food before it is eaten, and many cases of food poisoning are caused by faulty food handling and preparation. The risk of food poisoning can be reduced by attention to food hygiene.

Food intoxication

Some foods contain natural toxins which can be injurious to health. These include oxalic acid, solanine, aflatoxins and haemagglutinins.

Table 4.1   Food poisoning organisms.

Name	Symptoms	Incubation period	Typical foods affected
Bacillus cereus	Nausea, vomiting, diarrhoea, abdominal pain	1–16 hours	Rice dishes, custard, sauces
Campylobacters	Diarrhoea, fever, abdominal pain	1–7 days	Untreated milk, unchlorinated tap water
Clostridium botulinum	Difficulty in swallowing and breathing, double vision; fatal in 1–8 days	12–36 hours	Canned or vacuum-packed foods, raw fish
Escherichia coli	Abdominal pain, diarrhoea	12–24 hours	Sandwiches, salads, undercooked chicken or beefburgers
Listeria	Flu-like symptoms, fever, miscarriage, meningitis	5–30 days	Untreated milk, soft mould-ripened cheese (e.g. Brie, Camembert, Danish Blue), soft-whip ice cream from machines
Salmonellas	Diarrhoea, abdominal pain, fever	12–24 hours	Meat, meat products, poultry, eggs, milk and milk products
Staphylococci	Vomiting, abdominal pain	1–6 hours	Untreated milk, custard, cream, cold desserts, poultry, fish, meat

Oxalic acid

Oxalic acid is found in a number of fruits and vegetables, particularly rhubarb and spinach. Oxalic acid interferes with calcium absorption by forming an insoluble complex with calcium in the gut. However, rhubarb and spinach are good sources of non-starch polysaccharides (NSP), vitamins and minerals, and if people enjoy these foods they should be encouraged to eat them. Eating rhubarb and spinach two or three times a week is unlikely to cause harm to health.

Solanine

Solanine is found in green or sprouting potatoes. It causes diarrhoea and gastrointestinal discomfort and can be fatal.

Cutting off the green or sprouting portion is not enough because the toxin may also be found in the middle of the potato. Potatoes should be bought in quantities that can be consumed fairly quickly, and stored in a cool, dry place.

Aflatoxin

Some moulds can produce aflatoxin, a toxin that is known to induce liver cancer. Production of aflatoxin is a risk where dry foods are badly stored, and nuts and cereals are particularly susceptible. Stringent quality control tests reduce the risk of such foods being imported into the UK, and the chance of consuming aflatoxins in pre-packed nuts is small. The risk is greater with nuts bought in their shells.

Haemagglutinins

These toxins are found in red kidney beans but they are destroyed by thorough cooking. The consumption of uncooked red kidney beans can cause diarrhoea and sickness, and in some cases can be fatal because of damage to the red blood cells. Red kidney beans should always be soaked overnight, rinsed and boiled rapidly in fresh water for at least 20 minutes. Slow cookers do not always destroy the toxins because the temperature reached is not high enough. Soya beans contain similar toxins and should be pre-boiled before cooking. Other pulses should be cooked thoroughly but do not need to be pre-boiled.

Food hygiene

Attention to food hygiene reduces the risk of food poisoning. Safe food preparation involves common sense, including the following general guidelines:

Food purchase

- Choose foods processed for safety, e.g. always buy pasteurised and not untreated milk.
- Check date marks on food and use within the recommended period.
- Put chilled and frozen food into a refrigerator as quickly as possible.

Food preparation

- Wash hands thoroughly before food preparation, after every interruption and after handling raw foods such as meat, fish and poultry.
- Cover cuts and grazes on the hands with bandages or plasters.
- Keep all kitchen surfaces and all cooking equipment scrupulously clean.
- Avoid putting cooked or ready-to-eat food on surfaces which have been used for raw meat or poultry.
- Wash fruit, vegetables and salad in clean running water.
- Change dish cloths and tea towels every day.
- Keep pets away from food, work surfaces and dishes.
- Use separate knives for raw meat, cooked food and fresh vegetables.
- Use the refrigerator or microwave for thawing food.
- Do not refreeze raw food which has been thawed, or refreeze cooked food once thawed.

Food cooking

- Thaw pieces of frozen meat, fish and poultry thoroughly before cooking otherwise heating may not cook the centre enough; some of these foods can be cooked from frozen, but those which are bulky (e.g. joints) must be thawed.
- Cook food thoroughly, so that the temperature at the centre of the food reaches at least 70°C for at least 2 minutes; a thermometer can be used to check the temperature at the centre.
- Reheat cooked food thoroughly so that the temperature of the centre reaches 70°C.
- Never reheat cooked food more than once.
- Follow microwave instructions on food labels carefully.
- Follow all cooking times on food labels and recipes carefully.
- Avoid recipes which require raw egg such as mayonnaise, mousses or egg drinks.

Food storage

- Maintain refrigerators below 5°C and freezers below −18°C and defrost regularly.
- Do not overload refrigerators and freezers.
- Follow instructions for freezing on food labels.
- Store raw meat and poultry separately from other foods; in the refrig-

erator they should be below cooked foods and dairy products to avoid drips from raw meat.
- Do not put warm food in refrigerators and freezers.

Additives

Additives are deliberately added to food during processing to improve the taste, smell, texture and keeping qualities of food; they are not contaminants. The use of additives increases the variety of food and allows the transport of food in bulk.

Additives are also added to drugs, and pharmacists are often asked about this. A list of common prescription and OTC medicines which contain additives can be found in the National Pharmaceutical Association's information leaflet, 'Colourants in Oral Liquid Medicines' and further information can be obtained directly from the manufacturer.

Classification

Additives can be classified into the following major categories:

- Colours and flavours, which help to ensure uniformity in colour and flavour from batch to batch.
- Preservatives, which prevent microbiological spoilage, protecting against food poisoning and prolonging shelf life.
- Antioxidants, which prevent the oxidation of fat soluble vitamins and fats and oils going rancid; they also prevent enzyme browning of fruit, vegetables and juices, thus extending their keeping qualities
- Emulsifiers and stabilisers enable the mixing of ingredients that would normally separate.

In addition there are other categories of additives, such as anti-foaming agents which prevent scum formation and frothing, flavour modifiers which enhance or reduce the flavour of a food, and humectants which help to stop foods drying out.

Controls

Additives used in the UK must go through strict safety checks in order to be approved. There are over 300 listed additives (see Table 4.2) and they can be either natural or synthetic. Most of the additives are designated with a number, and those which are accepted as safe by the European Union also have an E in front of the number. Flavourings are exempt from these regulations and have no E number' all that is required by law is that 'flavouring' is added to the list of ingredients on the label.

Table 4.2   Food additives approved for use in the UK.

Colours
E100	curcumin
E101	riboflavin
101(a)	riboflavin-5'-phosphate
E102	tartrazine
E110	sunset yellow FCF
E120	cochineal
E122	carmoisine
E123	amaranth
E124	ponceau 4R
E127	erythrosine
E128	red 2G
E129	allura red AC
E131	patent blue V
E132	indigo carmine
E133	brilliant blue FCF
E140	chlorophyll
E141	copper complexes of chlorophyll and chlorophyllins
E142	green S
E150a	plain caramel
E150b	caustic sulphite caramel
E150c	ammonia caramel
E150d	sulphite ammonia caramel
E151	brilliant black PN, black PN
E153	carbon black (vegetable carbon)
E154	brown FK
E155	brown HT (chocolate brown HT)
E160(a)	alpha-carotene; beta-carotene; gamma-carotene
E160(b)	annatto; bixin; norbixin
E160(c)	capsanthin; capsorubin
E160(d)	lycopene
E160(e)	beta-apo-8'-carotenal
E160(f)	ethyl ester of beta-apo-8'-carotenoic acid
E161(b)	lutein
E161(g)	canthaxanthin
E162	beetroot red (betanin)
E163	anthocyanins
E170	calcium carbonate
E171	titanium dioxide
E172	iron oxides; iron hydroxides
E173	aluminium
E174	silver
E175	gold
E180	litholrubine BK

Preservatives
E200	sorbic acid
E202	potassium sorbate
E203	calcium sorbate
E210	benzoic acid
E211	sodium benzoate
E212	potassium benzoate

Cont.

Table 4.2   Cont.

E213	calcium benzoate
E214	ethyl 4-hydroxybenzoate (ethyl para-hydroxybenzoate)
E215	ethyl 4-hydroxybenzoate, sodium salt (sodium ethyl para-hydroxybenzoate)
E216	propyl 4-hydroxybenzoate (propyl para-hydroxybenzoate)
E217	propyl 4-hydroxybenzoate, sodium salt (sodium propyl para-hydroxybenzoate)
E218	methyl 4-hydroxybenzoate (methyl para-hydroxybenzoate)
E219	methyl 4-hydroxybenzoate, sodium salt (sodium methyl para-hydroxybenzoate)
E220	sulphur dioxide
E221	sodium sulphite
E222	sodium hydrogen sulphite (sodium bisulphite)
E223	sodium metabisulphite
E224	potassium metabisulphite
E226	calcium sulphite
E227	calcium hydrogen sulphite (calcium bisulphite)
E228	potassium bisulphite
E230	biphenyl (diphenyl)
E231	2-hydroxybiphenyl (orthophenylphenol)
E232	sodium biphenyl-2-yl oxide (sodium orthophenylphenate)
E233	2-(thiazol-4-yl) benzimidazole (thiabendazole)
E234	nisin
E235	natamycin
E239	hexamine (hexamethylenetetramine)
E242	dimethyl discarbonate
E249	potassium nitrite
E250	sodium nitrite
E251	sodium nitrate
E252	potassium nitrate
E280	propionic acid
E281	sodium propionate
E282	calcium propionate
E283	potassium propionate
E284	boric acid
E285	sodium tetraborate (borax)
E1105	lysozyme

Antioxidants

E300	L-ascorbic acid
E301	sodium L-ascorbate
E302	calcium L-ascorbate
E304	6-O-palmitoyl-L-ascorbic acid (ascorbyl palmitate)
E306	extracts of natural origin rich in tocopherols
E307	synthetic alpha-tocopherol
E308	synthetic gamma-tocopherol
E309	synthetic delta-tocopherol
E310	propyl gallate
E311	octyl gallate
E312	dodecyl gallate
E315	erythorbic acid
E316	sodium erythorbate

Cont.

Table 4.2   Cont.

E320	butylated hydroxyanisole (BHA)
E321	butylated hydroxytoluene (BHT)

Emulsifiers and stabilisers

E322	lecithins
E400	alginic acid
E401	sodium alginate
E402	potassium alginate
E403	ammonium alginate
E404	calcium alginate
E405	propane-1, 2-diol alginate (propylene glycol alginate)
E406	agar
E407	carrageenan
E407a	processed euchema
E410	locust bean gum (carob gum)
E412	guar gum
E413	tragacanth
E414	gum arabic (acacia)
E415	xanthan gum
E416	karaya gum
E417	tara gum
E418	gellan gum
E432	polyoxyethylene (20) sorbitan monolaurate (Polysorbate 20)
E433	polyoxyethylene (20) sorbitan mono-oleate (Polysorbate 80)
E434	polyoxyethylene (20) sorbitan monopalmitate (Polysorbate 40)
E435	polyoxyethylene (20) sorbitan monostearate (Polysorbate 60)
E436	polyoxyethylene (20) sorbitan tristearate (Polysorbate 65)
E440	pectins: pectin; amidated pectin
E442	ammonium phosphatides
E444	sucrose acetate isobutyrate
E445	glycerol esters of wood rosins
E460	microcrystalline cellulose; alpha-cellulose (powdered cellulose)
E461	methylcellulose
E463	hydroxypropylcellulose
E464	hydroxypropylmethylcellulose
E465	ethylmethylcellulose
E466	carboxymethylcellulose, sodium salt (CMC)
E470a	sodium, potassium and calcium salts of fatty acids
E470b	magnesium salts of fatty acids
E471	mono- and diglycerides of fatty acids
E472(a)	acetic acid esters of mono- and diglycerides of fatty acids
E472(b)	lactic acid esters of mono- and diglycerides of fatty acids
E472(c)	citric acid esters of mono- and diglycerides of fatty acids
E472(d)	tartaric acid esters of mono- and diglycerides of fatty acids
E472(e)	mono- and diacetyltartaric acid esters of mono- and diglycerides of fatty acids
E472(f)	mixed acetic and tartaric acid esters of mono- and diglycerides of fatty acids
E473	sucrose esters of fatty acids
E474	sucroglycerides
E475	polyglycerol esters of fatty acids

Cont.

Table 4.2 Cont.

E476	polyglycerol esters of polycondensed fatty acids of castor oil (polyglycerol polyricinoleate)
E477	propane-1,2-diol esters of fatty acids
E481	sodium stearoyl-2-lactylate
E482	calcium stearoyl-2-lactylate
E483	stearyl tartrate
E491	sorbitan monostearate
E492	sorbitan tristearate
E493	sorbitan monolaurate
E494	sorbitan mono-oleate
E495	sorbitan monopalmitate

Sweeteners

E420	sorbitol; sorbitol syrup
E421	mannitol
E953	isomalt
E965	maltitol; maltitol syrup
E966	lactitol
E967	xylitol
E950	acesulfame K
E951	aspartame
E952	cyclamic acid
E954	saccharin and its sodium, potassium and calcium salts
E957	thaumatin
E959	neohesperidine DC

Others

Acids, anti-caking agents, anti-foaming agents, bases, buffers, bulking agents, firming agents, flavour modifiers, flour bleaching agents, flour improvers, glazing agents, humectants, liquid freezants, packaging gases, propellants, release agents, sequestrants and solvents

E170	calcium carbonate; calcium hydrogen carbonate
E260	acetic acid
E261	potassium acetate
E262	sodium acetate; sodium hydrogen diacetate
E263	calcium acetate
E270	lactic acid
E290	carbon dioxide
E296	malic acid
E297	fumaric acid
E325	sodium lactate
E326	potassium lactate
E327	calcium lactate
E330	citric acid
E331	sodium dihydrogen citrate (monosodium citrate); disodium citrate; trisodium citrate
E332	potassium dihydrogen citrate (monopotassium citrate); tripotassium citrate
E333	monocalcium citrate; dicalcium citrate; tricalcium citrate
E334	L-(+)-tartaric acid
E335	monosodium L-(+)-tartrate; disodium L-(+)-tartrate

Cont.

Table 4.2   Cont.

E336	monopotassium L-(+)-tartrate (cream of tartar); dipotassium L-(+)-tartrate
E337	potassium sodium L-(+)-tartrate
E338	orthophosphoric acid (phosphoric acid)
E339	sodium dihydrogen orthophosphate; disodium hydrogen orthophosphate; trisodium orthophosphate
E340	potassium dihydrogen orthophosphate; dipotassium hydrogen orthophosphate; tripotassium orthophosphate
E341	calcium tetrahydrogen diorthophosphate; calcium hydrogen orthophosphate; tricalcium diorthophosphate
E350	sodium malate; sodium hydrogen malate
E351	potassium malate
E352	calcium malate; calcium hydrogen malate
E353	metatartaric acid
E354	calcium tartrate
E355	adipic acid
E356	sodium adipate
E357	potassium adipate
E363	succinic acid
E380	triammonium citrate
E385	calcium disodium ethylenediamine-$NNN'N'$-tetra-acetate (calcium disodium EDTA)
E422	glycerol
E431	polyoxyethylene (40) stearate
E450(a)	disodium dihydrogen diphosphate; trisodium diphosphate; tetrasodium diphosphate; dipotassium diphosphate; tetrapotassium diphosphate; dicalcium diphosphate; calcium dihydrogen diphosphate
E451	pentasodium triphosphate; pentapotassium triphosphate
E452	sodium polyphosphate; potassium polyphosphate; sodium calcium polyphosphate; calcium polyphosphates
E479b	thermally oxidised soya bean oil interacted with mono- and diglycerides of fatty acids
E500	sodium carbonate; sodium hydrogen carbonate (bicarbonate of soda); sodium sesquicarbonate
E501	potassium carbonate; potassium hydrogen carbonate
E503	ammonium carbonate; ammonium hydrogen carbonate
E504	magnesium carbonate; magnesium hydrogen carbonate
E507	hydrochloric acid
E508	potassium chloride
E509	calcium chloride
E511	magnesium chloride
E512	stannous chloride
E513	sulphuric acid
E514	sodium sulphate; sodium hydrogen sulphate
E515	potassium sulphate; potassium hydrogen sulphate
E516	calcium sulphate
E517	ammonium sulphate
E520	aluminium sulphate
E521	aluminium sodium sulphate
E523	aluminium ammonium sulphate
E524	sodium hydroxide

Cont.

Table 4.2   Cont.

E525	potassium hydroxide
E526	calcium hydroxide
E527	ammonium hydroxide
E528	magnesium hydroxide
E529	calcium oxide
E530	magnesium oxide
E535	sodium ferrocyanide
E536	potassium ferrocyanide
E538	calcium ferrocyanide
E541	sodium aluminium phosphate
E551	silicon dioxide (silica)
E552	calcium silicate
E553(a)	magnesium silicate synthetic; magnesium trisilicate
E553(b)	talc
E554	aluminium sodium silicate
E555	potassium aluminium silicate
E556	aluminium calcium silicate
E559	aluminium silicate (kaolin)
E570	stearic acid
E574	gluconic acid
E575	D-glucono-1,5-lactone (glucono delta-lactone)
E576	sodium gluconate
E577	potassium gluconate
E578	calcium gluconate
E620	L-glutamic acid
E621	sodium hydrogen L-glutamate (monosodium glutamate; MSG)
E622	potassium hydrogen L-glutamate (monopotassium glutamate)
E623	calcium dihydrogen di-L-glutamate (calcium glutamate)
E624	monoammonium glutamate
E625	magnesium diglutamate
E627	guanosine 5'-disodium phosphate (sodium guanylate)
E630	inosic acid
E631	inosine 5'-disodium phosphate (sodium inosinate)
E632	dipotassium inosinate
E633	calcium inosinate
E634	calcium 5'-ribonucleotide
E635	sodium 5'-ribonucleotide
E640	glycine and its sodium salt
E900	dimethylpolysiloxane
E901	beeswax
E902	candelilla wax
E903	carnauba wax
E904	shellac
E912	montan acid esters
E914	oxidised polyethylene wax
E920	L-cysteine hydrochloride
E925	chlorine
E926	chlorine dioxide
E927b	carbamide
E938	argon
E939	helium
E941	nitrogen

Cont.

Table 4.2   Cont.

E942	nitrous oxide
E948	oxygen
E953	isomalt
E999	quillaia extract
E1200	polydextrose
E1201	polyvinylpyrrolidone
E1202	polyvinylpolypyrrolidone
E1404	oxidised starch
E1410	monostarch phosphate
E1412	distarch phosphate
E1413	phosphated distarch phosphate
E1414	acetylated starch
E1422	acetylated distarch adipate
E1450	starch sodium octenyl succinate
E1505	triethyl citrate
E1518	glyceryl triacetate (triacetin)-Propan-1,2-diol (propylene glycol)

Food additives must be listed on food labels by category together with the serial number or chemical name, or both. There are other food additives approved for use in the UK which have not been assigned a serial number; these must be listed on food labels by chemical name.

Numbers prefixed with an E have also been approvd by the European Union.

Not all foods need to be labelled with a list of ingredients, and this means that additives are not always identified. Alcoholic drinks and chocolate may all contain additives but they do not appear on the label.

Some products appear with the statement 'free from artificial additives', but E numbers will appear on the label. This is because not all additives are synthetic and the product may contain natural ones.

Adverse effects

Additives have received a great deal of adverse publicity in the media so that many people believe they are unsafe. Some additives do cause adverse reactions in a few susceptible people but this is not nearly such a widespread problem as people think. The risks associated with high fat intake are probably about 100 times as great as those associated with additives. People who must avoid a specific additive should know both its name and number because either may appear on the food label.

Colours

Artificial colours have been associated with urticaria, asthma, purpura, severe abdominal cramps, vomiting and hyperactivity in children. The most common culprits are those which contain an azo group in their chemical structure. These include tartrazine (E102), sunset yellow (E110), carmoisine (E122), amaranth (E123), ponceau 4R (E124), red 2G (E128), black PN (E151), brown FK (E154) and brown HT (E155).

Preservatives

Preservatives, particularly benzoic acid and sulphites, have been implicated in asthma and chronic urticaria. Benzoic acid can be eliminated from the diet by avoiding foods containing E210–E219 and sulphites by avoiding those containing E221–E227.

Antioxidants

The antioxidants BHA (E320) and BHT (E321) have been associated with urticaria and hyperactivity in children and are often avoided in the dietary treatment of these conditions.

Monosodium glutamate (MSG)

MSG has long been used as a flavour enhancer in Oriental foods and has been implicated in the so-called Chinese Restaurant Syndrome which leads to facial flushing, headache and faintness in some individuals after eating Chinese food.

Contaminants

Pesticides

The term 'pesticide' includes several substances including insecticides, fungicides, weedkillers, soil sterilisers, rodent poisons, plant growth regulators and food storage protectors. The main reasons for using pesticides are to minimise losses of food and to prevent spoilage, and to take much of the risk out of farming. Without pesticides food would be much less varied and more expensive.

The levels of pesticides in food are monitored by the government. Only approved pesticides can be used in the UK and their use is restricted to specific applications and limited levels. Legal limits are set on the amount of pesticide that can be left on crops, and misuse of pesticides can result in prosecution.

Animal medicines and hormones

Levels of antibiotics and other medicines used in veterinary practice are tightly controlled. Many people are still concerned about hormones in meat but their use has been illegal throughout the European Union since 1988.

Organic produce

Concern about the effects of pesticide and drug residues in food has led to a demand for organically produced food. Organic foods are produced without the use of pesticides or other chemicals. However, it is difficult to avoid the effects of pollution or chemical sprays from a neighbouring farm or garden. Some organic foods have been shown to contain pesticide residues. Organic food cannot be said to be any healthier than food produced by the usual methods, but organic farming is kinder to the environment.

Organic foods are now controlled by the United Kingdom Register of Organic Food Standards (UKROFS). The following organisations are registered with UKROFS and may be used on organic food labels. These are the Soil Organisation, Organic Farmers and Growers, Bio-Dynamic Agricultural Association, Organic Food Manufacturers Federation and Scottish Organic Producers Association.

Further reading

Useful leaflets

Food Sense: a series of booklets entitled *Food Sense*; *Food Safety*; *About Food Additives*; *Understanding Food Labels*; *Food Protection*; *Healthy Eating*. Ministry of Agriculture, Fisheries and Food. (These can be obtained free of charge from Food Sense, London SE99 7TT.)

Section 3
Diet in Disease and Illness

Chapter 5
Disorders of the Cardiovascular System

Coronary heart disease

Definition

Coronary heart disease (CHD) is a term that covers a group of diseases, including angina pectoris and myocardial infarction (heart attack). These conditions are the result of two major processes, atherosclerosis and thrombosis.

Atherosclerosis is a long-term process in which there is an accumulation of fatty deposits in the lining of the arteries. By contrast thrombosis is a more acute vent which results in the formation of a thrombus or clot. The thrombus forms on the surface of the heart or blood vessel, and if the vessel is already narrowed by atherosclerosis the thrombus will block the vessel.

Incidence

Coronary heart disease continues to be a major cause of death in Britain although mortality rates have fallen in recent years. More men are prone to the disease than women and it is estimated that about one in five men suffers a heart attack before the age of 65 years. Risk of coronary heart disease in women increases after the menopause.

There are marked regional variations in the incidence of the disease in Britain with the highest incidence in the North of England, Scotland and Northern Ireland. Risk of heart disease is also higher in lower socio-economic groups.

Risk factors

The three classic risk factors for coronary heart disease are raised serum cholesterol, cigarette smoking and hypertension. Other risk factors include family history, being male, advancing age, diabetes mellitus, insufficient exercise, stress and socio-economic status, and also obesity – particularly when fat accumulates around the abdomen. Ethnic group is also important – Asians living in the UK have particularly high rates of CHD. Risk factors have a cumulative effect, so a middle-aged, overweight man who smokes will have a greater chance of developing coronary heart disease than a young, slim woman who does not smoke. Current research is looking at other factors, including those which influence the coagulability of the blood (e.g. fibrinogen), and also levels of homocysteine (which is influenced by folic acid intake), so the risk factor profile is likely to change.

The role of cholesterol

Cholesterol is an essential substance in the human body. It is a component of cell membranes and is needed for the body's manufacture of steroid hormones, vitamin D and bile salts. About 75% of the daily requirement is made in the liver and the remainder is obtained from the diet. Production in the liver normally responds to dietary intake so that if intake increases internal synthesis decreases.

Lipid metabolism

Fat from the diet enters the bloodstream mainly in the form of triglycerides and cholesterol. Triglycerides and cholesterol are insoluble in water and must be transported in plasma bound to specific proteins. The resulting complexes are called lipoproteins and comprise the following:

- Chylomicrons which carry dietary cholesterol and triglycerides to the peripheral tissues.
- Very low density lipoproteins (VLDL) which carry triglyceride produced by the liver to the peripheral tissues. Most of the serum triglyceride is in the form of VLDL. A high level of VLDL is associated with a high risk of coronary heart disease.
- Intermediate density lipoproteins (IDL) which are transient particles derived from the breakdown of VLDL. Some IDL is taken up by the liver and some is converted to low density lipoprotein.
- Low density lipoprotein (LDL) which is derived from VLDL and carries cholesterol from the liver to the peripheral tissues. LDL gives up some of its cholesterol to the fatty deposits in the arterial walls, and high levels of LDL are associated with a high risk of coronary heart disease.
- High density lipoproteins (HDL) which carry excess cholesterol from the peripheral tissues to the liver for disposal. Elevated levels of HDL are therefore thought to be protective.

Disorders of lipid metabolism

Disorders of lipid metabolism may be classified as primary or secondary. Primary hyperlipidaemias are caused by an inherited defect in lipid metabolism, and secondary hyperlipidaemias may be caused by disease, such as diabetes mellitus, renal failure, gout or hypothyroidism, or by excessive alcohol intake and obesity. The administration of some drugs (see Chapter 26) may also lead to hyperlipidaemia.

Primary hyperlipidaemias have been classified in several ways and the classification system is still evolving. The European Atherosclerosis Society classifies hyperlipidaemia according to concentrations of total cholesterol and triglyceride in the blood, while the Fredrickson/WHO classification gives a more detailed assessment of the lipoproteins that are elevated. It is now also possible to classify some hyperlipidaemias according to cause. Features of hyperlipidaemias are summarised in Table 5.1.

Table 5.1 Types of primary hyperlipidaemias.

Type	Serum cholesterol	Serum triglyceride	Lipoproteins	Causes
Familial hypercholesterolaemia	Raised	Normal	LDL	Caused by abnormal or decreased LDL receptors
Familial chylomicronaemia	Normal or slightly raised	High	Chylomicrons	Lipoprotein lipase deficiency which breaks down chylomicrons
Familial combined hyperlipidaemia	Raised	Raised	LDL and VLDL	Increased production of VLDL in the liver leading to increased secretion of LDL
Familial hypertriglyccridaemia	Slightly raised	Raised	VLDL and chylomicrons	Increased production of triglyceride resulting in increased secretion of VLDL

Primary hyperlipidaemias are rare, but because blood cholesterol levels are so high the risk of coronary heart disease may be very great. Patients with primary hyperlipidaemias have physical signs, including lipid deposits under the skin (xanthomata), as well as signs of coronary heart disease in early life.

Dietary influences and coronary heart disease

There is still a great deal of debate about the influence of diet on coronary heart disease. Diet is not itself a risk factor, but components of diet can alter other risk factors such as serum cholesterol, hypertension, diabetes mellitus and obesity.

Dietary factors discussed include the different types of fatty acids (i.e. saturated, polyunsaturated and monounsaturated), cholesterol, complex carbohydrates and anti-oxidant nutrients.

Saturated fatty acids

The dietary factor most commonly associated with raised serum cholesterol is saturated fat, and many studies have shown a strong positive relation between saturated fat intake and incidence of coronary heart disease. However, not all saturated fatty acids raise serum cholesterol levels. Only myristic and palmitic acids do this. These acids are found in milk and dairy produce, meat and meat products, coconut, some margarines, and baked cereal products. Shorter chain and longer chain saturates do not have this effect.

Polyunsaturated fatty acids

For many years polyunsaturated fatty acids mainly of the n-6 series have been synonymous with lipid lowering, but increasing the intake of polyunsaturates is now thought to be less important than reducing that of saturated fat. While n-6 polyunsaturates reduce the level of LDL cholesterol, they also reduce the level of HDL cholesterol which protects against coronary heart disease. Very high intake of polyunsaturates may also increase the risk of cancer.

The Inuit, who have a diet high in total fat and also in the n-3 poly-unsaturated fatty acids, have low rates of coronary heart disease. The n-3 polyunsaturates do not lower serum cholesterol levels, but they do lower elevated serum triglyceride levels and reduce blood clotting.

Monounsaturated fatty acids

Populations in some Mediterranean countries have a high intake of mono-unsaturated fatty acids (mainly in the form of olive oil) and have low rates of heart disease. However, Mediterranean diets differ in a number of other important respects, such as greater fruit and vegetable consumption. There is currently insufficient evidence to recommend an increase in monounsaturates in the UK diet.

Trans fatty acids

Trans fatty acids, formed by the partial hydrogenation of vegetable oils to produce margarine and vegetable shortening, increase the ratio of LDL to HDL in the blood. Increasing consumption of these fatty acids may contribute to the occurrence of CHD.

Dietary cholesterol

In the majority of people, dietary cholesterol has little influence on serum cholesterol levels. Saturated fatty acids have a much greater effect. A cholesterol-lowering diet should not be confused with a low cholesterol diet.

Complex carbohydrates

A high intake of complex carbohydrates is associated with a low incidence of coronary heart disease, but there is no evidence that this is a direct effect of the carbohydrate. Diets high in complex carbohydrates are often low in fat, and this is likely to be the more important factor.

Non-starch polysaccharides (dietary fibre)

Low rates of CHD have also been linked to diets high in NSP, but it is difficult to evaluate the importance of NSP in a diet which is also likely to be low in fat. Soluble NSP does have an independent cholesterol-lowering influence, but the amounts required to achieve a measurable effect are quite large (e.g. 100 g of oats a day).

Anti-oxidant nutrients

Epidemiological studies have shown that high blood levels of anti-oxidants (eg vitamins C, E, and beta-carotene) and a high intake of fruit and vegetables are linked with a reduced risk of CHD. Evidence is also emerging that vitamin E at higher intakes than can be obtained from the diet may be protective. Flavonoids, another group of compounds with anti-oxidant activity, are found widely in fruit and vegetables and also in tea. Several studies have suggested a role for flavonoids in the prevention of CHD, but the effects of individual flavonoids have not yet been fully elucidated.

Folic acid

There is growing evidence that elevated plasma levels of homocysteine, a metabolite of the amino acid methionine, may be an additional risk factor for CHD. Homocysteine may act by generating free radicals which oxidise LDL, cause damage to the arteries and influence the development of atherosclerosis.

Low blood levels of folic acid are often associated with high blood homocysteine levels and there is some experimental evidence that by increasing dietary intake of folic acid and possibly vitamins B_6 and B_{12}, blood concentrates of homocysteine can be reduced.

Alcohol

Heavy alcohol consumption increases the risk of CHD, probably because of an associated increase in blood pressure. Moderate alcohol consumption seems to decrease the risk, and this may be due to an influence of clotting factors in the blood or to an increase in the level of HDL cholesterol in the blood which is thought to be protective. It does not seem to matter what type of alcohol is consumed, and despite the media attention given to red wine, it cannot be stated categorically that red wine is more beneficial than beer or other alcoholic drinks.

Drinking water

Populations who live in areas of hard drinking water seem to have a lower risk of CHD than those who live in soft water areas. This may be due to the higher content of minerals, particularly calcium and magnesium.

Coffee

An association between drinking coffee and coronary heart disease is suspected. Current evidence indicates that it is the method of preparation rather than the intake of caffeine which is important. Boiled coffee appears to be more closely linked with CHD than instant or filtered coffee.

Dietary supplemenjts

There are a number of dietary supplements which make claims about their ability to prevent CHD, but they should not be used as substitutes for reducing other risk factors.

Fish oil and fish liver oil capsules are now widely promoted for the prevention of CHD. There is some scientific basis for this because they are rich in n-3 polyunsaturates. Pharmacists should, however, explain the dangers of fat-soluble vitamin toxicity if recommended doses of fish liver oils are exceeded.

Garlic is thought to protect against CHD but the evidence so far is inconclusive and a beneficial dose has not been identified.

Nicotinic acid, one of the metabolites of the B-vitamin niacin, is prescribable for lipid lowering, but it should not be sold as a dietary supplement for this purpose. It can cause unpleasant side-effects, particularly in high dosage.

Magnesium supplements are promoted for the prevention of CHD. Consumption of hard water, which is rich in magnesium and other minerals, has been associated with a reduced risk of CHD. Intravenous magnesium may help to prevent secondary heart attacks in patients who have already had one, but these findings do not justify the recommendation of oral magnesium supplements for prevention of CHD.

Oat bran is available for sprinkling on food and adding to cooking. Oat bran is rich in soluble NSP which is thought to be beneficial in lowering blood cholesterol levels.

Reducing risk factors

Many people visit community pharmacies years before they develop CHD, and pharmacists have a useful role in explaining risk factors, persuading individuals to lose weight and to stop smoking and discouraging high alcohol intake. Dietary advice based on healthy eating guidelines (see Chapter 3) can also be given as the opportunity arises.

Cholesterol measurement is becoming increasingly common, and pharmacists may be asked for advice by patients who have had serum cholesterol measured. It should be remembered that measurement of blood cholesterol is just one aspect of screening for CHD risk, and measurement of blood pressure, body weight and smoking history are just as important.

Guidelines for patient counselling on serum cholesterol levels have been published by the European Atherosclerosis Society and adapted for the pharmacy (see Table 5.2). These guidelines are the best available at the moment, but they are based on somewhat arbitrary cut-off points and the optimum cholesterol level is considered to be 5.2 mmol/litre. The problem is that about 60% of the UK population have higher levels than this, and obsession with cholesterol numbers may cause the public a great deal of anxiety. Pharmacists should therefore use these guidelines with care and be aware that they are likely to develop and change as knowledge grows.

Table 5.2 Guidelines for patient counselling in relation to serum cholesterol levels.

< 5.2 mmol/litre	Explain that the level falls within desirable limits. Question the patient about other risk factors, e.g. smoking and exercise, and counsel on healthy lifestyle including diet
5.2–6.5 mmol/litre	Explain that the level is a little higher than desirable but normal for the UK. Give dietary advice and counsel about other risk factors. Advise repeat measurement in 6 months' time
6.5–7.8 mmol/litre	Explain that the level is above normal range. Counsel about other risk factors and refer to GP unless patient has already had specialist advice
< 7.8 mmol/litre	Explain that the level is too high. Counsel about other risk factors and refer to GP unless patient has already had specialist advice. The condition can be inherited, so first-degree relatives should also be tested.

Adapted from King, M.J. and Blenkinsopp, A. (1989) *Pharmaceutical Journal* **243**, 736–40.

Patients who have had their serum cholesterol measured outside the pharmacy are likely to have already received advice about lifestyle, including diet. If such advice has been given by another health professional, particularly a dietitian, the role of the pharmacist is to confirm it and to encourage the patient to adhere to the diet.

Dietary advice for lipid lowering

Dietary advice for lowering blood cholesterol is basically the same as that for current healthy eating but certain aspects of diet should be emphasised. These are fat and NSP, particularly soluble NSP. Body weight should be reduced if appropriate.

Fat

The aim is to reduce fat intake towards 30% of total energy intake. This can be achieved by increasing the intake of starchy carbohydrates and reducing the intake of foods high in fat (see Chapter 3).

The type of fat is also important, and saturated fat should be reduced. While increasing the intake of n-6 polyunsaturates is not considered to be as important now as formerly, it may be useful in slim patients liable to lose weight if they reduce total fat intake. Substituting a polyunsaturated margarine for butter may be useful in patients who do not need to lose weight. In those who do need to lose weight a low fat spread is a better choice.

Increasing the intake of n-3 polyunsaturates may help to lower serum triglyceride levels and prevent blood clotting, which may assist in preventing heart attacks. Polyunsaturates of the n-3 series are found principally in fatty fish such as tuna, pilchards, whitebait, trout, sardines, mackerel and herring. Patients with raised blood cholesterol can be advised to eat a serving of fatty fish two or three times a week.

Increasing the intake of monounsaturates does not appear to increase blood cholesterol level and may help to lower it. Monounsaturated fat (e.g. olive oil) may therefore be used with polyunsaturated fat to replace saturated fat in the diet.

Soluble NSP

Diets high in NSP-rich carbohydrates are often low in fat. It is therefore useful advice to increase the intake of NSP. There are two types of NSP, soluble and insoluble, and it is soluble NSP which appears to have the most effect on lowering blood cholesterol levels. Soluble NSP is found in foods such as oats and oat products (e.g. muesli), pulses (eg dried peas, dried beans and lentils) and in fruit and green leafy vegetables.

Summary of dietary advice for lowering blood cholesterol.

(1) Reduce and maintain body weight in the ideal range
(2) Reduce fat (particularly saturated fat) intake
(3) Increase the intake of soluble NSP
(4) Eat fatty fish (e.g. sardines, tuna, herring, mackerel) two or three times a week

---

More details of practical guidelines for making these dietary changes can be found in Chapter 3.

Hypertension

It is difficult to define hypertension for individuals in Britain because, in common with other Western countries, blood pressure increases with age. The current recommendations of the British Hypertension Society are that when:

- The initial blood pressure is systolic $\geqslant$ 160mmHg or diastolic $\geqslant$ 100mmHg, these values are sustained on repeat measurement
- The initial blood pressure is systolic 140–159mmHg or diastolic is 90–99mmHg and the patient has a $\geqslant$ 15% risk over 10 years of coronary heart disease or end-organ damage (e.g. left ventricular hypertrophy, renal impairment), treat if these values are sustained on repeat measurement
- The initial blood pressure is systolic 140–159mmHg or diastolic 90–99mmHg and the patient has a < 15% risk over 10 years of coronary heart disease and no end-organ damage, reassess annually and discuss lifestyle changes
- The initial blood pressure is systolic < 140mmHg and diastolic < 90mmHg, reassess in 5 years and discuss lifestyle changes

The joint recommendations advise a target systolic blood pressure of less than 140mmHg and diastolic of less than 85mmHg, but the targets in diabetes are lower (130/80mmHg).

Dietary management

Attention to diet as well as other lifestyle factors, such as stress and smoking, is important in the management of hypertension, even for those patients who are treated with anti-hypertensive drugs. The most important dietary factors are obesity, alcohol, sodium and potassium.

Obesity

Weight should certainly be reduced and maintained within the ideal range (see Chapter 19). Weight loss often results in a significant fall in blood pressure.

Alcohol

Patients with hypertension should limit alcohol, ideally to one unit a day for women and two units a day for men (for an explanation of alcohol units see Chapter 3).

Sodium

High sodium intake has been linked with hypertension but only some individuals are susceptible. Currently there is no way of identifying who these people are, but, since most people consume more sodium than they need, it is advisable to reduce salt intake. Salt should be avoided or reduced in cooking and at the table, and the intake of foods high in sodium (see Table 3.4) should be restricted to two or three portions a week.

Sodium is also found in several medicines, particularly in antacids and effervescent preparations (see Tables 5.3 and 5.4). High sodium preparations should also be avoided by patients with heart failure and renal failure, during pregnancy and by those taking lithium.

Table 5.3   Low sodium antacids (< 1 mmol/tablet or 10 ml dose).

Actonorm gel	Gelusil tablets
Algicon suspension	Maalox suspension
Altacite tablets	Maalox Plus tablets
Altacite suspension	Maalox Plus suspension
Alu-Cap	Maalox TC tablets
Asilone liquid	Maalox suspension
Asilone tablets	Mucogel suspension
Asilone suspension	Topal tablets
Dijex tablets	Unigest tablets
Dijex liquid	

Table 5.4   High sodium antacids.

Product	Sodium content
Alka-Seltzer tablets	22 mmol/tablet
Bismag tablets	2 mmol/tablet
Bisodol powder	7 mmol/g
De Witts powder	7 mmol/g
Eno's powder	8 mmol/g
Gastrocote tablets	1 mmol/tablet
Gaviscon Advance	4.6 mmol/10 ml
Gaviscon tablets	2 mmol/tablet
Gaviscon liquid	3 mmol/10 ml
Gaviscon 250 tablets	1 mmol/tablet
Infant Gaviscon	1 mmol/sachet
Magnesium trisilicate mixture	6 mmol/10 ml
Magnesium trisilicate powder	3 mmol/g
Roter tablets	2 mmol/tablet
Soda Mint tablets	4 mmol/tablet
Sodium bicarbonate	12 mmol/g

Potassium

Diets low in sodium are often high in potassium and vice versa, but potassium may have a separate blood pressure lowering effect.

Potassium is widely distributed in food including fruit, especially bananas, apricots, rhubarb, blackcurrants, dried fruit and fruit juices. It is also found in vegetables, particularly pulses and potatoes, wholegrain cereals, milk and dairy products, fish and meat. Potatoes are a particularly useful source of potassium if the patient cannot afford to buy fruit.

Salt substitutes

Several pharmacies stock salt substitutes (e.g. Lo-salt, Ruthmol and Selora) which are low in sodium and high in potassium. Salt substitutes are not suitable for everybody. Patients who are taking ACE inhibitors (e.g. captopril), potassium-sparing diuretics (e.g. amiloride) or cyclosporin, or those who have renal disease, should not use them without referral to the GP. This is because of a risk of potassium toxicity.

Calcium

There is a suggestion that low calcium intake is linked with hypertension, and some studies have shown that calcium supplementation could lower blood pressure. If calcium does have an effect, patients on anti-hypertensive drugs should not take calcium supplements without referral to the GP in case blood pressure control is altered.

Lifestyle advice

Stress and smoking exacerbate hypertension. Patients should therefore be advised to reduce stress wherever possible and stop smoking. Physical exercise is also important.

Further reading

British Nutrition Foundation (1997) *Diet and Heart Disease. A Round Table of Factors*, 2nd edn. Chapman and Hall, London.

Department of Health (1994) *Nutritional aspects of cardiovascular disease. Report on Health and Social Subjects No 46*. HMSO, London.

National Heart Forum (1997) *At Least Five a Day. Strategies to Increase Fruit and Vegetable Consumption*. The Stationery Office, London.

National Heart Forum (1997) *Preventing Coronary Heart Disease. The Role of Antioxidants, Vegetables and Fruit*. The Stationery Office, London.

National Heart Forum (1999) *Looking to the Future. Making Coronary Heart Disease an Epidemic of the Past*. The Stationery Office, London.

Useful addresses

British Heart Foundation, 14 Fitzhardinge Street, London W1H 4DH. Tel: 0207 935 0185.

The Stroke Association, Stroke House, Whitecross Street, London EC1Y 8JJ. Tel: 0207 566 0300.

Coronary Prevention Group, Plantation House, 31–35 Fenchurch Street, London EC3M 3NW. Tel: 0207 628 4844.

Chapter 6
Diabetes Mellitus

Diabetes mellitus is caused by a deficiency in insulin or a diminished effectiveness in its utilisation. If insulin is lacking or is used ineffectively, levels of glucose in the blood rise, and once the renal threshold is exceeded glucose is excreted in the urine.

Symptoms

Impaired glucose utilisation leads to increase in urine output, thirst, weight loss and a sense of fatigue. Blood cholesterol levels are often raised in diabetes, and patients have an increased risk of coronary heart disease.

Classification of diabetes mellitus

There are two types of diabetes mellitus, type 1 or insulin dependent diabetes (IDDM0, and type 2 or non-insulin dependent diabetes (NIDDM).

Type 1 diabetes usually develops during the first 30 years of life but can occur at any age. This type of diabetes is treated with insulin and a controlled diet.

Type 2 diabetes develops more commonly in middle-aged people who are overweight or obese. Some cultural groups such as Asians and Afro-Caribbeans have a greater risk of developing the disease. Type 2 diabetes may be treated by diet alone. If this proves unsuccessful, control may be achieved by the use of diet, oral hypoglycaemics, and sometimes insulin.

Risk factors

The risk of developing diabetes appears to be related to genetic factors, stress and infection, but it may arise as a result of disorders such as pancreatic disease, and endocrine conditions such as hyperthyroidism.

No single dietary factor can be said to cause diabetes, but there is certainly a close association between obesity and type 2 diabetes. Thus any type of diet which leads to obesity may increase the risk of developing type 2 diabetes.

Dietary management

Diet plays a crucial role in the management of both types of diabetes mellitus but advice has changed considerably since the early 1980s. The traditional diabetic diet, which emphasised the importance of carbohydrate restriction, was relatively high in fat and may have increased the risk of coronary heart disease to which patients with diabetes are particularly prone.

The current guidelines of the British Diabetic Association are shown in the box below. They are similar to the general healthy eating guidelines for the adult population, and emphasise the importance of a diet high in complex carbohydrates, low in fat and low in sugar. For diabetics who are part of a household or family, this means that they do not need a significantly different diet from everyone else. Any sense of isolation is therefore minimised.

Recommendations of the British Diabetic Association for patients with diabetes mellitus (1992).

(1) Reduce and maintain body weight in the ideal range
(2) Complex carbohydrates should make up 50–55% of the dietary energy intake
(3) Sugar is allowed up to 25 g a day provided that it is part of a diet low in fat and high in NSP and that it is consumed as part of a meal
(4) NSP intake should be about 18 g a day (equivalent to 30 g of dietary fibre), concentrating on soluble NSP
(5) Fat intake should not exceed 30% of energy intake and saturated fat should not exceed 10% of energy intake
(6) Cholesterol intake should not exceed 300 mg a day
(7) Protein intake should comprise about 10–15% of energy intake
(8) Salt intake should be limited to 6 g a day

Initial dietary advice should be given by a dietitian. The role of the pharmacist is to confirm such advice, give encouragement and make sure that the patient is adhering to the diet. Even though the diabetic diet is now little different from the diet which all healthy adults should be eating, many patients find it difficult to comply with the recommendations.

Dietary advice given to patients with type 1 diabetes is generally similar to that given to patients with type 2 diabetes although the advice given to individual patients may differ. Distribution of carbohydrate intake throughout the day is usually more important in type 1 diabetes, but dose and type of insulin preparation should also be adjusted to suit the individual patient's lifestyle.

The main aims in the dietary management of diabetes are:

- To reduce weight in the overweight patient and maintain optimum weight
- To maintain blood glucose levels as near to normal as possible, preventing both hypoglycaemia and hyperglycaemia
- To maintain blood lipid levels as near normal as possible.

The main factors to consider in the diabetic diet are body weight, the amounts and types of carbohydrate and fat in the diet and the level of alcohol consumption.

Body weight

The most important factor in dietary management is the achievement of ideal body weight. Not all patients need to lose weight but many do. It is important to realise that, by achieving weight loss, patients may not need any other treatment. For patients on oral hypoglycaemic drugs, weight reduction may often mean that the dose can be reduced or the drug stopped altogether.

Carbohydrate

At least half of the dietary energy should be obtained from carbohydrate, and the type of carbohydrate is important. The recommendation for patients with diabetes is that most of the carbohydrate should come from starchy, complex sources, preferably those rich in non-starch polysaccharides (NSP). Soluble NSP has a beneficial effect on blood lipid levels, lowering both total and LDL cholesterol. Sugar need no longer be eliminated from the diet but it should be restricted.

Sugar

The British Diabetic Association recommends that sugar intake should be limited to 25 g a day and that it should only be consumed as part of a whole meal of snack. Sugar consumed as part of a meal has less of an effect on blood glucose level than sugar consumed on its own. Thus, a small amount of jam on wholemeal bread is an acceptable snack whereas a few boiled sweets on their own is not.

Sugar in drinks should be avoided. If sweetness is desired, an energy-free sweetener (e.g. aspartame, acesulfame K or saccharin – see Chapter 19) should be used. Sweeteners providing energy, such as fructose, sorbitol and maltodextrin, should be restricted.

Care with sugar intake does not just mean the obvious sources such as sugar in drinks, jam and confectionery. A common error made by patients is to assume that natural fruit juices, honey and reduced-sugar products are low in sugar. Such misconceptions should be corrected.

Fat

The diabetic diet should be low in fat because of the risk of cardiovascular complications. A low fat diet will also help the overweight patient to reduce body weight. However, there is increasing debate regarding the most beneficial balance between carbohydrate and fat in the diabetic diet. Diets which are very low in fat (eg 20–25% of dietary energy) may increase serum triglycerides, reduce HDL cholesterol, and increase postprandial glucose and insulin levels without lowering LDL cholesterol. These changes have been linked with an increased risk of coronary artery disease in some people with diabetes. For this reason, investigators are looking at the effects of monounsaturated fats instead of carbohydrates to compensate for restricted saturated fat in the diet and to avoid the adverse effects of high carbohydrate diets. It is likely, therefore, that when the British Diabetic Association guidelines for the diabetic diet are updated, the recommendation will be made that patients be evaluated on an individual basis with nutritional advice based on specific abnormalities and treatment goals. The concept of a single diabetic diet is not appropriate.

Alcohol

Complete avoidance of alcohol is unnecessary but diabetic patients should be aware of the energy content of alcoholic drinks, particularly if weight reduction is necessary. One pint of beer provides about 756 kJ (180 kcal) and a glass of wine about 420 kJ (100 kcal).

Alcohol also produces hypoglycaemia, particularly if consumed on its own, so, like sugar, alcohol should always be consumed as part of a meal. Patients with diabetes should ideally not exceed an alcohol limit of one unit a day (for an explanation of alcohol units, see Chapter 3). They should certainly not drink and drive.

Alcohol may interact with tolbutamide to cause an unpleasant flushing reaction and is best avoided by patients taking this drug. Other oral hypoglycaemics do not have this effect and, within the restrictions discussed above, these patients may safely drink alcohol.

Diabetic foods

Diabetic foods such as chocolate, sweets, cakes, biscuits and jams have been available for many years but are now sold in very few pharmacies. They were designed in the 1960s when sugar restriction was considered to be essential, but now that complete exclusion of sugar is not required, patients may eat small amounts of ordinary chocolate, biscuits and jams.

Most diabetic foods provide slightly, but not substantially, less energy than comparable non-diabetic products but many have a higher fat content. The greatest difference between diabetic and non-diabetic foods is the sugar content; sweeteners such as sorbitol and fructose are used to replace the sugar in diabetic products.

Products which do not offer a 50% saving in total energy must be labelled 'Not suitable for the overweight diabetic'. Products containing a sugar substitute which contributes to energy intake, such as fructose or sorbitol, must be labelled 'Best eat less than 25 g a day of (name of substitute)'. One reason for the 25 g limit is that such sugar substitutes are usually eaten as part of a high-calorie food such as chocolate, and it is sensible to limit total intake of such foods. Another factor is that some sugar substitutes, particularly sorbitol, can have a laxative effect when consumed in large quantities.

There are now many low sugar/low energy fizzy drinks, fruit squashes, fruits tinned in natural juice and reduced-sugar jams on the market. Such foods are usually lower in energy and cheaper than their diabetic counterparts and are a better choice for patients with diabetes.

Patients with diabetes should be discouraged from thinking that their diet is 'different' but that it is a pattern of healthy eating which most people should be following. The existence of diabetic foods creates the impression that a 'different' diet and 'special' foods are necessary. In addition, some patients believe that diabetic products can be eaten as 'extras' in unlimited quantities in addition to their ordinary diet. Pharmacists should certainly correct this misconception.

Diet in other cultural groups

There is a greater incidence of diabetes in some cultural groups in the UK (e.g. Asians and Afro-Caribbeans). The traditional diets of these groups of people can fulfil the recommendations for people with diabetes but there may be some problems with fat intake (e.g. from ghee in Asian diets and coconut in Afro-Caribbean diets). Greater problems probably occur when traditional diets are altered as a result of settling in the UK (see Chapter 23).

Hypoglycaemia

Hypoglycaemia is a common complication of diabetes mellitus, particularly in those patients treated with insulin and occasionally in those treated with oral hypoglycaemics. Hypoglycaemia can occur at any time of the day or night and may be caused by:

- Delayed or missed meals
- Too large a dose of insulin or oral hypoglycaemics
- Strenuous activity without taking extra carbohydrate beforehand
- Drinking large amounts of alcohol, particularly on an empty stomach

Symptoms of hypoglycaemia vary from one person to another but common warning sighs include sweating, trembling, pallor, palpitations, weakness and feelings of hunger. Shortage of glucose may also affect brain function resulting in lack of concentration, forgetfulness, irritability, unsteadiness, aggressive or irrational behaviour and ultimately fits and unconsciousness as the blood sugar continues to fall.

As soon as a patient feels the warning symptoms of hypoglycaemia, some form of fast-acting sugar should be taken immediately. This could be either:

- Three or four lumps of sugar
- Two or three glucose tablets
- A glass of a sugary drink such as Lucozade, fruit squash or non-diet fizzy drink
- Four or five sweets of the type which can be quickly chewed (*not* boiled sweets)

This should be followed by some slow-acting carbohydrate food to prevent the blood sugar falling again. Most patients will know from experience what they need, but suggestions include:

- Two digestive biscuits
- One slice of bread or a bread roll
- One fruit yoghurt
- One portion of fruit

If the patient becomes unconscious, it is important to remember that no food or fluid should be given by mouth because this may cause choking. The patient may be treated by a doctor who can give an intravenous injection of glucose. Alternatively a glucagon injection may be given by a person (often a relative of the patient) who has been trained to use it, or the sugar-gel preparation (Hypostop) may be squeezed between the cheeks and gums. Sugar is absorbed into the bloodstream from this preparation without the need to swallow.

If the patient suffers from severe or frequent attacks of hypoglycaemia the doctor should be notified.

Exercise

Patients with diabetes should be encouraged to take regular exercise just the same as everyone else. Exercise may reduce insulin requirements and can sometimes improve overall glucose tolerance. Patients who are poorly controlled should, however, avoid strenuous exercise until control is improved.

Type 1 diabetes

In type 1 diabetes, alterations in carbohydrate intake and insulin dose will be required before the start of the activity. Exercise increases the uptake of glucose by the muscles and therefore acts in the same way as an extra dose of insulin. The main danger of exercise is hypoglycaemia, and this can be avoided either by eating some extra carbohydrate or by reducing the dose of the preceding insulin injection or sometimes both.

The extra carbohydrate may be eaten as part of the last meal before the exercise. More bread, potatoes, yoghurt or fruit juice or a mixture of such foods will normally be sufficient. If exercise is taken more than 2–3 hours after a meal, a quick snack in the form of biscuits, cereal bars, yoghurt or fruit should be consumed just beforehand. Carbohydrate top-ups may also be required during exercise, particularly if the activity is prolonged. These could include glucose tablets, chocolate bars or fruit juice.

If the dose of insulin is reduced before exercise, care should be taken not to reduce it too much because of increasing the risk of hyperglycaemia.

Most patients learn by experience what is right for them in terms of the amount of extra carbohydrate and reduction in insulin dose, and initial advice should always be given by the diabetic clinic.

Type 2 diabetes

People who are managed by diet or diet with metformin do not usually need to take any special precautions before exercise. Patients taking sulphonylurea drugs including chlorpropamide, glibeclamide, gliclazide, glipizide, gliqui-done, tolazamide and tolbutamide do need to take special precautions, because administration of these drugs can lead to low blood sugar during exercise. Risk of hypoglycaemia may be minimised either by eating extra carbohydrate before the exercise or by reducing the dose of the previous tablet.

Patients should be encouraged to discuss details of drug administration and diet at the diabetic clinic.

Illness

During times of illness, diabetic control is likely to worsen and extra care must be taken with carbohydrate intake. In insulin dependent diabetes care should also be taken with insulin dose. Even if the patient cannot eat normally, the usual dose of insulin is still required and sometimes more.

A satisfactory blood glucose level can be maintained by replacing normal meals with food and drinks which supply about 10 g of carbohydrate every hour (see Table 6.1). In very nauseated patients a few mouthfuls of sweet drink should be given about every 20 minutes.

If oral rehydration solutions are required, advice should be given about their glucose content (see Table 6.2).

Diabetes and coeliac disease

Patients suffering from both diabetes mellitus and coeliac disease are not unknown, and the demands of a gluten-free diet must then be met in addition to the recommendations for diabetes. Patients will need specialist guidance from a dietitian. One of the difficulties is that, in avoiding gluten, patients may consume high fat foods and increase the risk of coronary heart disease. Patients with diabetes already have an increased risk of CHD.

Pharmacists may advise such patients about the range of gluten-free cereals and breads which are low in fat and rich in complex carbohydrates. Many of these products are available on prescription (see Table 9.5).

Table 6.1 Foods suitable for use in patients who feel ill (each item contains 10 g carbohydrate).

3 tablespoons (50 ml) Lucozade
1 small glass (100 ml) unsweetened fruit juice
1 small glass (100 ml) cola
1 large glass (200 ml) milk
Half a sachet of Build-Up
3 teaspoons Complan
2 teaspoons Horlicks, Ovaltine or drinking chocolate
100 ml canned tomato soup
200 ml canned cream soup, e.g. chicken, mushroom
1 scoop (50 g) of ice cream
1 digestive biscuit
1 fruit yoghurt
3 glucose tablets
3 sugar lumps
2 teaspoons of jam, honey or marmalade

Table 6.2 Glucose content of oral rehydration solutions.

Product	Glucose content/sachet or tablet
Diocalm Junior (Seton Scholl)	4 g
Dioralyte (Rhone-Poulenc Rorer)	
Tablets	1.62 g
Powder	3.56 g
Electrolade (Eastern)	4 g
Rehidrat (Searle)	4.09 g (plus sucrose 8.07 g, fructose 0.7 g)

Useful addresses

British Diabetic Association, 10 Queen Anne Street, London W1M 0BD. Tel:0207 323 1531.
Diabetes Foundation, 177a Tennison Road, London SE25 5NF. Tel:0208 656 5467.

Chapter 7
Cancer

Cancer is now the leading cause of death in Britain. Despite the advances made in diagnosis and treatment, one in four deaths in Britain is due to cancer.

This chapter will discuss two aspects of dietary advice in cancer, that is, advice which may help to reduce the risk of developing cancer, and advice which may help patients who already have it.

Reducing the risk of cancer

Risk factors

The most important risk factor for lung cancer is, of course, smoking, which is thought to be responsible for about 30% of cancer deaths. Certain occupational exposures such as asbestos and gamma radiation can interact additively with smoking.

Exposure to sunlight is the most important factor for skin cancer.

Dietary influences

Diet is thought to have a role in the development of about one-third of cancers, but identifying components of diet which could increase or decrease the risk is remarkably difficult.

Fat

High fat diets are associated with an increased risk of cancers at various sites including the colon, breast and prostate. Fat is the most energy-dense component of the diet and high fat diets increase the risk of obesity. High fat diets can therefore directly increase the risk of those cancers that are influenced by obesity – e.g. endometrial cancer. The type of fat is also important. Populations consuming large amounts of saturated fat appear to be at increased risk of cancer. High intake of polyunsaturated fat may also increase the risk of cancer by causing damage to cell membranes through the production of free radicals. However, an adequate intake of anti-oxidant nutrients (e.g.

beta-carotene, selenium and vitamins C and E) helps to prevent damage to cell membranes caused by free radicals.

Fruits and vegetables

Increasing fruit and vegetable intake is associated with reduced incidence of cancer at almost every site. Fruits and vegetables are rich in the anti-oxidant nutrients, and while the evidence does not yet warrant a recommendation for dietary supplements containing these nutrients, it does emphasise the importance of fruits and vegetables in the diet.

Complex carbohydrates

Low intakes of complex carbohydrates are associated with cancer of the colon. The initial suggestion that this was an effect of low intake of non-starch polysaccharides seemed likely but has not been proven. Diets high in NSP often contain large quantities of fruit and vegetables and are also low in fat. It is the overall pattern of the diet which is likely to be more important than NSP per se.

Meat

High meat intake has been linked with cancer, particularly of the colon, but also possibly of the breast, pancreas, prostate and lung. However, diets that contain a lot of meat may also be high in fat and protein and it is difficult to separate these different influences. The cooking process may also be important. Studies which have shown a positive relationship between meat intake and cancer have often involved grilled and barbecued meat. Hetero-cyclic amines are produced in relatively large amounts in meats cooked in these ways and these compounds have been shown to be mutagenic and carcinogenic in animals.

   A recent report from the Committee on Medical Aspects of Food and Nutrition Policy recommended that lowered consumption of red meat and processed meat would probably reduce the risk of colon cancer, particularly in people who eat large quantities of these meats. However, because meat is a good source of other nutrients such as iron and zinc, care should be taken to replace it with other nutrient-dense foods such as wholegrain cereals and fruit and vegetables.

Alcohol

Heavy alcohol consumption is associated with cancers of the mouth, larynx, oesophagus and liver.

Smoked, cured and salt-preserved foods

Oesophageal and stomach cancers are linked with diets containing large amounts of smoked and salt-preserved foods. The smoke for curing appears to produce carcinogens in the food, and salt-preserved foods contain nitrites which can be transformed into nitrosamines. Nitrosamines can be carcinogenic in the stomach.   ᵖᵍ 14 ,ᵖᵍ 15

Grilling foods over open flames, particularly to the point of charring, may also lead to the production of carcinogenic substances on the surface of foods, and charring of foods should be avoided.

Obesity

Obesity is associated with increased risk of cancer of the endometrium and prostate and post-menopausal breast cancer.   ᵖᵍ 5

Dietary advice for reducing cancer risk

Dietary advice for reducing the risk of cancer is summarised below:

> (1) Reduce fat intake, both saturated and unsaturated
> (2) Eat at least five servings of fruit and vegetables every day
> (3) Increase the intake of starchy carbohydrates, particularly those rich in NSP
> (4) Moderate alcohol intake
> (5) Avoid becoming overweight
> (6) Consume salt-cured, salt-pickled and smoked foods in moderation
> (7) Avoid charred food

Lifestyle advice

The risk of developing cancer can be reduced by not smoking, avoiding excessive exposure to the sun and following safety instructions when handling any substance which may cause cancer.

Treatment of cancer

Cancer may be treated by surgery or radiotherapy or with drugs.

Dietary management

Both the nature of the disease and the treatment are likely to lead to nutritional problems. Dietary management will depend on the severity of the disease, and some patients will need enteral or parenteral feeding (see Chapters 28 and 29), particularly if they are unable to eat or if they have had intestinal surgery. In these cases the supervision of a dietitian is essential.

For patients who are able to eat normally, the best advice is to eat a healthy and well balanced diet. This is just as important for patients with cancer as for healthy people.

Eating difficulties

Some patients may find that they cannot eat normally because of the side-effects of radiotherapy or chemotherapy. If this is a long-term problem, the advice of a dietitian is essential. A multivitamin and mineral supplement may be required either because the patient is not eating normally or because there is a risk of nutrient deficiency due to the drug treatment.

Nausea and vomiting are common side-effects of chemotherapy, and patients may find the following advice useful:

- Eat small, frequent meals rather than three large meals
- Eat bland foods such as bread, toast, crackers, scrambled eggs and potatoes which are less likely to induce nausea than spicy or fatty food
- Avoid the smell of cooking food
- Drink fluid in between meals rather than with meals to prevent feeling too full.

Advice for patients with sore mouths or difficulty in swallowing can be found in Chapter 28.

Complementary diets

There is no need to follow a special diet unless prescribed by a dietitian, but many people choose to follow a complementary diet when they have cancer because they feel that they are helping themselves in a positive way.

Patients are often attracted to complementary diets because of the unpredictable cure rate for the disease and because of the potential for unpleasant side-effects from the treatment. Not surprisingly, alternative therapies abound. None has any proven therapeutic benefit, but they can offer psychological benefit by making patients feel more involved in their own care.

The Bristol Diet is perhaps one of the most well known of the complementary diets and is now much less restrictive than it used to be. The diet is based on whole, fresh foods with a strong emphasis on raw fruit and vegetables.

Patients should always be referred to a dietitian before embarking on any complementary diet because the diet may be too restrictive, so increasing the risk of nutritional deficiency.

Dietary supplements

Vitamin and mineral supplements are often advocated both to prevent and to cure cancer. There is little evidence to support any of these claims. However, patients with cancer may not be able to meet nutritional requirements from food alone, and a multivitamin and mineral supplement could be useful.

Further reading

Department of Health (1998) *Nutritional aspects of the development of cancer. Report on Health and Social Subjects No 48.* The Stationery Office, London.

World Cancer Research Fund and American Institute for Cancer Research (1997) *Food, Nutrition and the Prevention of Cancer: a Global Perspective.*

Useful addresses

British Association of Cancer United Patients (BACUP), 3 Bath Place, Rivington Street, London EC2A 3JR. Tel: 0800 181199 or 0207 613 2121.

Cancer Care Society, 21 Zetland Road, Redland, Bristol BS6 7AH. Tel: 0117 942 7419.

Cancer and Leukaemia in Childhood Trust (CLIC), CLIC Annexe, 3 Nugent Hill, Cotham, Bristol BS6 5TD. Tel: 0117 924 8844.

Cancerlink (telephone helpline), 17 Britannia Street, London WC1X 9JN. Tel: 0207 833 2451.

Cancer Relief Macmillan Fund, Anchor House, 15–19 Britten Street, London SW3 3TZ. Tel: 0207 351 7811.

Cancer Research Campaign, 10 Cambridge Terrace, London NW1 4JL. Tel: 0207 224 1333.

Malcolm Sargent Cancer Fund for Children, 14 Abingdon Road, London W8 6AF. Tel: 0207 937 4548.

Chapter 8
Gastrointestinal Disease

This chapter discusses the dietary management of gastrointestinal disorders which may present in community pharmacies. These include dental caries, dyspepsia, gastro-oesophageal reflux duseuse, peptic ulcer, diarrhoea, constipation, haemorrhoids, irritable bowel syndrome, diverticular disease, Crohn's disease, ulcerative colitis, cystic fibrosis and the problems faced by patients with stomas.

Dental caries

This is the progressive destruction of the tooth enamel. The development of dental caries requires three factors to be present. These are susceptible teeth, cariogenic bacteria and a substrate for such bacteria.

Nutrition and dental caries

Good nutrition is important during the period of tooth development, and the healthiest teeth develop when adequate supplies of all nutrients are available. Teeth start to develop before birth, and at this stage the mother's diet is particularly important.

Fluoride

The availability of fluoride during the period of tooth development confers considerable resistance to dental decay. Where the fluoride content of the drinking water is less than 700 µg per litre (0.7 parts per million), fluoride preparations are a suitable alternative. Information about the fluoride content of the local water supply can be obtained from the Water Company.

Fluoride tablets (En-De-Kay, Fluor-a-day, Fluorigard and Oral-B Fluoride) and drops (En-De-Kay and Fluorigard) are available. Patients should be advised to suck tablets or dissolve them in the mouth because the topical effect of fluoride is just as if not more important than the systemic effect.

Topical preparations such as fluoride mouthwashes (En-De-Kay and Fluorigard) and fluoride toothpaste are also useful. Mouthwashes can be used daily or weekly; daily use of a less concentrated rinse is more effective than weekly use of a more concentrated one. Gels are available but these

Table 8.1 Daily doses of fluoride (expressed as fluoride ion) in infants and children.

Fluoride content of water	Under 6 months	6 months–3 years	3–6 years	Over 6 years
< 300 µg	none	250 µg	500 µg	1 mg
300–700 µg	none	none	250 µg	500 µg
> 700 µg	none	none	none	none

[1] Recommended by the British Dental Association, the British Society of Paediatric Dentistry and the British Association for the Study of Community Dentistry.

should be applied under the supervision of a dentist. Less concentrated gels can be obtained for home use.

Sugar

All extrinsic (free) sugars have the potential to cause dental caries but sucrose is the worst culprit. It is the most commonly consumed sugar, and if cariogenic bacteria are present it is rapidly metabolised to produce acid. This lowers the pH surrounding the teeth, causing calcium to leave the tooth enamel, which starts the process of dental decay.

The physical form of sugar-containing foods is also important. Sticky foods such as toffees and sweets which adhere to the surface of the teeth do the most harm. This is because there is more time for the bacteria to metabolise them, resulting in a prolonged period of low pH, so allowing longer for demineralisation of the teeth.

The potential for tooth decay is also affected by the frequency of consumption of sugar. Eating sugar three or four times a day causes the pH to remain low for longer periods than if sugar is consumed only once a day. Sugar consumed as part of a meal has less cariogenic potential than sugar consumed on its own.

Pharmacists will be aware of the increasing availability of sugar-free medicines, and these are particularly important for patients who are taking a medicine for long periods of time. A list of sugar-free medicines is available from the National Pharmaceutical Association, and dietary guidelines to help prevent dental caries are given below.

Dietary advice to help the prevention of dental caries.

(1) Moderate sugar intake
(2) Avoid or reduce the intake of sticky foods
(3) Eat fruit, raw vegetables, bread or crackers as between-meal snacks instead of sweets
(4) Eat sugary foods as part or at the end of a meal instead of in between meals

Dyspepsia

Dyspepsia (indigestion) is a common symptom which may occur shortly after eating or drinking. In many instances it is unrelated to disease of the gastrointestinal tract and is caused by overeating and excessive drinking. In some patients dyspepsia may be due to reflux oesophagitis, hiatus hernia or peptic ulceration.

Dietary advice

Patients with dyspepsia need dietary advice based on common sense with no rigid rules. If the patient has been bolting meals or drinking too much alcohol, symptoms are likely to disappear when these habits are curtailed. Some patients may find that certain foods bring on their symptoms, so such foods should be avoided. All patients should be advised to stop smoking.

Gastro-oesophageal reflux disease

Gastro-oesophageal reflux occurs when there is regurgitation of the gastric and duodenal contents into the oesophagus. This causes inflammation and dyspepsia. Reflux oesophagitis may also be associated with hiatus hernia. It may be treated with antacids but the patient should always be offered lifestyle advice which includes diet.

Dietary advice

Gain in body weight will often aggravate dyspepsia, so overweight and obese patients should be advised to reduce their weight. Improvement in symptoms is often seen after relatively modest weight loss. Large amounts of food and drink are best avoided because of raising the intra-gastric pressure which tends to promote reflux. Eating just before bedtime should particularly be discouraged because this increases the amount of nocturnal acid secretion.

Foods and drinks which cause symptoms should be avoided, and the patient is usually the best judge of these. Fatty and spicy foods, chocolate, peppermint, coffee, alcohol and citrus fruits may induce reflux by lowering oesophageal sphincter tone, by irritation of inflamed oesophageal mucosa or by stimulating gastric acid secretion.

Apart from these specific dietary measures the diet should be based on healthy eating guidelines. Constipation should be avoided.

Lifestyle advice

Reflux oesophagitis commonly occurs after meals and may be aggravated by lying flat, stooping or bending. The head of the bed should be raised by about 20 cm, and tight clothes should be avoided. Smoking should be actively discouraged because it lowers oesophageal sphincter pressure and reduces the resistance of the gastric mucosa to acid.

> **Dietary advice for patients with reflux oesophagitis and hiatus hernia.**
>
> (1) Lose weight if necessary
> (2) Eat small meals at frequent and regular intervals
> (3) Avoid eating large meals or drinking large quantities of fluid
> (4) Avoid eating during the three hours before going to bed
> (5) Avoid food and drinks which cause symptoms

Peptic ulcer

Peptic ulcers are damaged areas of tissue developing in areas of the gastro-intestinal tract which are exposed to the irritant action of the gastric acid. They may occur in the lower oesophagus, the stomach and the duodenum. They are usually treated with drugs, and surgery is used less often than previously.

Dietary advice

There is a great deal of confusion amongst the general public about diet in peptic ulcer. Traditional advice to eat bland meals, such as boiled fish in milk, is not longer considered to be necessary. Patients have lived for years on such unappetising foods without any apparent benefit. Ulcer-healing drugs such as H_2-receptor antagonists and proton-pump inhibitors have revolutionised the treatment of ulcers and allow patients to eat a much more normal diet.

There is no need for a special diet, and patients should be advised to follow the general principles of healthy eating. The guidelines in the box below will not necessarily help to heal an ulcer but may help to alleviate the symptoms of dyspepsia. In addition, smoking must be stopped and medicines such as aspirin which irritate the stomach should be avoided.

> **Dietary advice for patients with peptic ulcer.**
>
> (1) Lose weight if necessary
> (2) Eat small meals at frequent and regular intervals
> (3) Avoid any food or drink which causes dyspepsia
> (4) Avoid strong coffee, tea and alcohol
> (5) Avoid fried and spicy food

Diarrhoea

Diarrhoea is an increase in the frequency and looseness of bowel movements. Acute diarrhoea is commonly caused by viral and bacterial infection of the gastrointestinal tract and may be a result of food poisoning (see Chapter 4) or change of location and climate, such as when travelling (see Chapter 22).

Acute diarrhoea generally lasts only for a few days and in otherwise healthy adults it is usually not serious. Chronic diarrhoea which lasts longer than a few days may be the result of a more serious underlying disorder, such as inflammatory bowel disease or bowel cancer.

Dietary advice in acute diarrhoea

The most important treatment for acute diarrhoea is the prevention or treatment of water and electrolyte depletion, particularly in babies, young children and frail elderly people who are at particular risk of dehydration. Antidiarrhoeal drugs should never be used as a substitute for oral rehydration therapy.

Intestinal absorption of sodium and water is enhanced by glucose so replacement of fluid and electrolytes is best achieved by use of a solution containing sodium, potassium and glucose. Patients with diabetes should be advised about the glucose content (see Table 6.3).

The best formulation for oral rehydration fluids is open to debate but a sodium ion content of 50–70 mmol/litre (Dioralyte, Electrolade and Rehidrat) may be the most beneficial for mild to moderate diarrhoeas. About one to two glassfuls (200–400 ml) should be drunk after every loose motion, or the solution may be sipped throughout the day. Extra drinks may also be consumed.

Fatty foods are best avoided during an acute attack of diarrhoea and should be reintroduced gradually. When the individual wants to start eating gain, foods to suggest include dry toast or crackers with thin soup or drinks made from meat or vegetable extract.

Whether patients should avoid milk or not is debatable, but if diarrhoea is prolonged there is a risk of lactose intolerance. This is because diarrhoea may lead to a deficiency of the enzyme lactase.

Constipation

Constipation may be defined as the difficult and infrequent passage of hard stools. Defaecation can vary between three times a week and three times a day, and it is when there is a reduction in frequency and increasing difficulty in passing stools that the individual is said to be constipated.

Dietary advice

Many cases of constipation can be treated by dietary measures, and the use of laxatives should not be encouraged. Daily exercise also helps to maintain regular bowel movements.

The intake of non-starch polysaccharides (NSP) should be increased, and the insoluble type of NSP is the most useful. Insoluble NSP is found principally in wholegrain cereals and wholemeal bread. Fluid intake should also be increased.

The practice of sprinkling bran on food should be discouraged, because raw bran is rich in phytate which may jeopardise absorption of some minerals and trace elements (e.g. zinc, copper, calcium). Mixed diets high in NSP are unlikely to have this effect.

Haemorrhoids (piles)

Haemorrhoids occur when the veins in the anus and rectum become enlarged or irritated. They are commonly caused by straining as a result of constipation, and they frequently occur in pregnancy.

Dietary advice

Dietary treatment involves the consumption of a diet high in NSP – particularly insoluble NSP – and drinking plenty of fluid. This helps to soften the stools and so prevent straining.

Flatus (wind)

Flatus is air or, more usually, a mixture of gases formed in the intestine and expelled through the anus. It is sometimes caused by dietary factors.

Dietary advice

Patients are sometimes the best judges of what causes their wind, and experimenting with the diet and reducing the intake of foods which appear to cause problems is often helpful. Pulses and other vegetables appear to be common culprits, but such foods should ideally form a part of a healthy diet so they should not be avoided altogether. It may help to increase the intake of pulses gradually, and if dried beans are used they must be soaked and cooked properly. If time is limited, canned beans are a useful alternative.

Fizzy drinks and chewing gum are best avoided, and patients should be advised to eat all food slowly and to try to relax at mealtimes.

Irritable bowel syndrome

Irritable bowel syndrome is a very common bowel disorder in which patients complain of either diarrhoea or constipation, or the two conditions may alternate. Chronic abdominal pain may or may not be present.

Dietary management

Increasing the intake of NSP has been regarded as the mainstay of dietary treatment for patients with irritable bowel syndrome, but patients with constipation are more likely to benefit than those with diarrhoea.

Some patients with diarrhoea-predominant irritable bowel syndrome may have food intolerance, and wheat and corn appear to be common culprits. Intolerances to tea, coffee, chocolate and dairy products have also been identified.

Many patients are ready to believe that food allergies are responsible for their symptoms. However, exclusion diets are not an easy option, and patients should be discouraged from trying them out for themselves. Close supervision by a dietitian is required to ensure that the diet remains nutritionally adequate.

Diverticular disease

Diverticular disease is common, particularly in people aged over 50. Straining to pass hard faeces may cause ruptures in the intestine which form pouches known as diverticuli. Patients may be asymptomatic but they may suffer from abdominal pain and altered bowel habit.

Dietary management

A diet high in NSP and an increase in fluid intake may be tried.

Crohn's disease

Crohn's disease is a chronic inflammatory disease which can affect any part of the gastrointestinal tract. It commonly starts in young adulthood. Symptoms include abdominal pain, diarrrhoea and loss of weight because nutrients are not properly absorbed. The activity of the disease varies, and sometimes patients are in relative remission.

Dietary management

The dietary management of Crohn's disease requires expert dietetic help because of the risk of nutrient deficiency which may arise as a result of malabsorption.

The most important aspect of dietary management in Crohn's disease is that the diet should be nutritionally adequate. Energy and vitamin and mineral supplements are sometimes prescribed by the dietitian or doctor. Patients may believe that certain foods are responsible for their symptoms, but care should be taken in excluding foods because of the risk of deficiencies.

During the active stage of the disease when the symptoms are particularly severe, patients may require enteral or parenteral nutrition. During remission, patients are often advised to eat a diet high in NSP, but this may not be suitable for patients with intestinal narrowing.

Ulcerative colitis

Ulcerative colitis is a chronic inflammatory disorder which affects only the large intestine. Like Crohn's disease it commonly starts in young adulthood.

Dietary management

When the disease is in an acute stage, enteral or parenteral feeding may be required. Patients who are in remission should be encouraged to eat a normal healthy diet, even one which is high in NSP. Vitamin and mineral supplements may be required but should be prescribed by a doctor. Although food intolerances may be responsible for symptoms, patients should be discouraged from eliminating foods from their diets without referral to a dietitian.

Cystic fibrosis

Cystic fibrosis is a genetically inherited disorder in which there is widespread malfunction of the exocrine glands. It is characterised by chronic respiratory tract disorders, and pancreatic enzyme deficiency leads to malabsorption of fat and other nutrients, particularly the fat-soluble vitamins.

Physiotherapy is an important part of management, and prophylactic administration of antibiotics may be considered necessary to prevent infection. Pancreatin preparations are used to compensate for reduced or absent exocrine section.

Dietary management

During the past few years there has been a change in thinking on what constitutes a healthy diet for patients with cystic fibrosis. Reduction in fat intake used to be emphasised, because with the older pancreatin preparations fat digestion was so poor. With the advent of the newer coated pancreatin preparations the dose can be adjusted to allow for adequate fat absorption, although fat restriction may be necessary in some patients.

Fat is a source of concentrated energy, and a normal intake is now recommended because of the high energy requirement of patients with cystic fibrosis. Patients must be encouraged to eat a diet which provides sufficient energy to maintain their weight in the ideal range. Most patients need at least 20% more energy (calories) than normal, but some may need 50% extra or even 100% more than normal. In practice this is likely to mean eating three main meals and two to three snacks daily. These should include liberal amounts of high energy foods, such as full fat milk, cheese, meat and eggs. Even butter and margarine and sugary foods may be encouraged because they are rich in energy. In patients with reduced appetite, high energy oral supplements or overnight artificial feeding may be necessary.

Malabsorption of food can lead to a wide range of nutritional deficiencies including vitamins and essential fatty acids. Routine vitamin supplements, especially of the fat-soluble vitamins, are prescribed by the doctor. Mineral supplements are sometimes needed, and salt supplements may be required but only during heatwaves or by patients who take vigorous exercise.

Stomas

Diet

Patients with colostomies and ileostomies should be encouraged to follow as normal a diet as possible, but many individuals find that their diet affects the timing, quantity and quality of their stoma output. Many patients with stomas restrict their diet to avoid excessive flatus, odour or fluidity in their stools, but foodstuffs should always be tried more than once and large numbers of foods, particularly fruit and vegetables, should not be excluded from the diet without referral to a dietitian. It is particularly important for patients with stomas to chew their food well. The box below gives some guidance on foods which may cause problems for patients with stomas.

Excessive flatus is caused by foods which are fermented in the proximal colon. Odour is therefore more of a problem for patients with transverse and descending colostomies than for those with ascending colostomies.

Patients with colostomies may occasionally become constipated and this is best treated by increasing the NSP content of the diet. The routine use of laxatives should be discouraged without referral to the GP.

Patients with ileostomies may have a reduced ability to absorb fluid and electrolytes, particularly during the first two months after surgery. Patients with ileostomies should be encouraged to drink an extra two to three glassfuls of fluid a day, and ensure adequate intake of sodium and potassium. Salt drinks such as Bovril, and potassium-rich drinks such as fruit juices, are useful for patients in the first months following an ileostomy operation.

Dietary guidelines for patients with ostomies.

Foods which may cause odour:
Cheese, eggs, fish, pulses, onions, cabbage

Foods which may cause wind:
Pulses, cabbage, onions, cucumbers, radishes, fizzy drinks, fatty foods, irregular meals

Foods which may cause loose bowels:
Green beans, broccoli, spinach, raw fruit, beer, highly spiced foods

Foods which may cause blockage:
Dried fruit, fruit and vegetable skins, nuts and seeds, citrus fruits, cabbage and celery

---

Further reading

British Nutrition Foundation (1999) *Oral Health. Diet and Other Factors.* Elsevier, Oxford.

Useful addresses

British Colostomy Association, 15 Station Road, Reading, Berks RG1 1LG. Tel: 0118 939 1537.

British Dental Health Foundation, Eastlands Court, St Peter's Road, Rugby CV21 3QP. Tel: 01788 546365.

British Fluoridation Society, Sandlebrook, Mill Lane, Alderley Edge, Cheshire SK9 7TY. Tel: 01565 873936.

Coeliac Society of the UK, PO Box 220, High Wycombe, Bucks HP11 2HY. Tel: 01494 437278.

Cystic Fibrosis Trust, 11 London Road, Bromley, Kent BR1 1B7. Tel: 0208 464 7211.

Ileostomy Association of Great Britain and Ireland, Amblehurst House, Black Scotch Lane, Mansfield, Notts NG18 4PF. Tel: 01623 280999.

National Association for Colitis and Crohn's Disease, 4 Beaumont House, Sutton Road, St Albans, Herts AL1 5HH. Tel: 01727 844296.

Urostomy Association, Buckland, Beaumont Park, Danbury, Essex CM3 4DE. Tel: 01245 224294.

Chapter 9
Food Intolerance

Food intolerance is a general term which describes an abnormal and repro-
ducible physiological response to an ingested food component, constituent or
additive. This chapter discusses food intolerance which is caused by allergy,
pharmacological substances, malabsorption and inborn errors of metabolism
(Fig. 9.1).

Food allergy

There has been widespread publicity given to 'food allergies', and people are
quick to believe that they or their children have them. Genuine food allergy is
in fact relatively rare, occurring in about 2% of the population. 'Food
allergy' is a term which should be reserved for adverse reactions to food

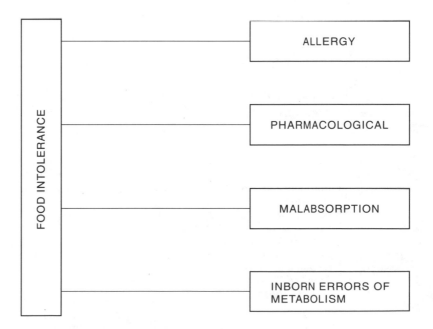

Fig. 9.1 Causes of food intolerance.

which involve the immune system and should not be confused with the broader term, 'food intolerance'.

Sufferers of true food allergy display altered or abnormal tissue reactions to some food molecules which act as antigens and cause the production of antibodies. The allergic reaction results from the combination of antigen and antibody.

Incidence

Food allergy may occur at any age but is most common in early childhood and tends to disappear spontaneously after the age of about 5 years. Where there is a family history of allergic reactions (e.g. asthma, eczema or hay fever), a child in the family is at increased risk of developing a food allergy.

Substances commonly associated with food allergy

The most common antigens are proteins, and foods to which patients are commonly allergic include milk, eggs, wheat, soya, nuts (especially peanuts), soft fruits (e.g. strawberries), fish and shellfish.

Milk protein

Cow's milk sensitivity occurs in between 0.5% and 7% of all babies. Symptoms may develop when an infant is transferred from breast to cow's milk. Alternatively, they may appear after 6 to 18 months of life.

Treatment involves the replacement of cow's milk by a milk substitute. Soya milk (e.g. Ostersoy) is commonly used although some babies also develop intolerance to soya protein. Hydrolysed protein formulas (e.g. Pregestimil) tend to be less allergenic and may be used as an alternative. Milk substitutes available on prescription for milk protein sensitivity are listed in Table 9.1.

Symptoms usually recede within 24–48 hours and the substitute milk may be recommended for periods of 6–12 months before a re-challenge with cow's milk. If the allergy is severe, avoidance of beef products may also be

Table 9.1 Products prescribable under Advisory Committee on Borderline Substances (ACBS) guidelines for milk protein sensitivity.

Milk formulae
Farley's Soya Formula (Farley)
Infasoy (Cow & Gate Nutricia)
Isomil (Abbott)
Nutramigen (Bristol-Myers)
Prosobee (Bristol-Myers)
Wysoy (Wyeth)

Foods
Comminuted chicken meat (Scientific Hospital Supplies)

necessary because the range of proteins present is similar to that in cow's milk.

In addition to dairy foods, milk products may be found in soups, gravy, low fat spreads, cakes, desserts, biscuits, rusks, infant foods, sauces, chocolates and sweets. Milk is not always an obvious ingredient so food labels should always be checked for the substances shown in Table 9.2. Milk-free infant foods are available and are labelled accordingly.

Table 9.2   Ingredients which indicate the presence of milk.

Calcium caseinate	Milk protein
Casein	Milk sugar
Caseinate	Skimmed milk
Demineralised whey	Sodium caseinate
Lactose	Whey
Milk	Whey protein

Parents should be discouraged from attempting to treat a suspected milk allergy themselves. Medical advice should always be sought before a cow's milk formula is abandoned. Some parents may try goat's or sheep's milk, but it should be stressed that these milks are low in certain nutrients, such as folic acid, and should not be used in young children.

Peanuts

Peanut allergy is particularly serious – indeed it can be life threatening. Peanuts and peanut oil are used in many foods, and labels should be studied carefully. Peanut oil is also found in some medicines. Sensitive individuals need to carry adrenaline (e.g. EpiPen) with them at all times and be instructed in advance how to use it. In addition, the packs need to be labelled so that, if the patient collapses, someone else can give the injection.

Additives

Food additives can occasionally cause adverse reactions which may be due to allergy (see Chapter 4).

Symptoms

The allergic response to a food can occur within a few minutes or be delayed for several hours. Immediate reactions include lip swelling, tingling of the mouth and throat, vomiting and rhinorrhoea. Asthma, conjunctivitis, urticaria and angio-oedema generally occur within an hour. Diarrhoea and bloating tend to occur later. All of these symptoms are transitory, and if the food is not eaten again they usually subside within 24 hours. Eczema, however, may take several days to develop.

Diagnosis

It is essential that allergy is properly diagnosed, and patients should be discouraged from making a self-diagnosis. Cases of suspected allergy should always be referred to the doctor.

Diagnosis of food allergy is easy when there is a characteristic early response to a food that is eaten occasionally, but it is more difficult if the clinical reaction is delayed. There are no straightforward tests for food allergy comparable to the urine glucose test for diabetes mellitus.

Skin tests are used in which small quantities of extracts containing suspected antigens are pricked or scratched into the skin. A well defined weal and area of redness within 20 minutes is taken as a positive response. The radioallergosorbent test (RAST) is a test designed to show the presence of specific IgE antibodies. Neither of these tests is particularly reliable so results should be interpreted with caution.

Another test involves the use of a small quantity of the suspected food hidden in a made-up dish so that patient are unaware that they are eating the food.

Elimination diets

If the food or foods can be identified and eliminated from the diet, the symptoms will not recur. If this is not possible, all the foods that commonly provoke allergic reactions are eliminated from the diet for 2 to 3 weeks. One food is then reintroduced into the diet every 3 to 7 days. Elimination diets carry a risk of nutrient deficiency, and individuals should be discouraged from trying them out without the supervision of a dietitian.

Pharmacological substances

Some constituents of food such as caffeine and histamine can have a pharmacological effect, particularly if ingested in large quantities.

Caffeine

Caffeine is found in tea, coffee and cola drinks, and in some individuals large intakes can provoke reactions such as sweating, palpitations, tremor and dyspepsia. Caffeine withdrawal may itself cause symptoms such as headache, depression and anxiety. Tea, coffee and cola drinks are available in decaffeinated forms.

Principal dietary sources of caffeine are shown in Table 9.3, but pharmacists should remember that many OTC analgesics and cold remedies contain caffeine in amounts ranging from 15 to 100 mg per dose.

Table 9.3 Caffeine content of some common foods and drinks.

Food	Approximate caffeine content (mg)
Coffee, ground (1 cup)	110
instant (1 cup)	65
Decaffeinated coffee (1 cup)	3
Tea (1 cup)	50
Decaffeinated tea (1 cup)	3
Drinking chocolate (1 cup)	5
Cola drink (1 can)	50
Decaffeinated cola (1 can)	3
Lucozade (1 glass)	40
Chocolate bar, dark, 100 g	40
milk, 100 g	20

Salicylates

Salicylates occur naturally in a wide range of foods and are present in high concentrations in herbs and spices. Some individuals are intolerant to salicylates (including aspirin), and this may be manifest as asthma, severe rhinitis, urticaria, and occasionally anaphylactic shock. Salicylates are excluded in the Feingold diet for the treatment of hyperactivity (see Chapter 17).

Vasoactive amines

Foods such as cheese, pickled fish, chocolate, citrus fruit, yeast extract and red wine or port contain pressor amines such as histamine, tyramine and serotonin and may provoke attacks of migraine in susceptible individuals. Lack of food may also provoke a migraine attack.

Patients who persistently have migraines after drinking red wine can be advised to try white wine instead. Red wine, strong beers, strong lagers and dark ales are most likely to provoke migraine attacks than white wine, pale lager and light ales. Individuals may also find that they suffer migraine more readily after brandy, whisky, dark rum, port and sherry than white spirits, such as vodka, gin and white rum.

Malabsorption

Malabsorption of nutrients may occur for a number of reasons, including enzyme deficiencies, reduction in absorptive surface of the intestine or infection. Only two disorders of malabsorption will be discussed: carbohydrate intolerance and coeliac disease.

Carbohydrate intolerance

Carbohydrate intolerance is commonly caused by a deficiency of one or more of the enzymes which split disaccharides into simple sugars. Disaccharides then enter the colon taking water with them, which may lead to osmotic diarrhoea. In the colon they are fermented causing flatulence, abdominal discomfort and cramp.

Lactose intolerance

Lactose intolerance is caused by a deficiency of the enzyme lactase, a condition which may be present from birth although this is relatively rare. Secondary lactose intolerance may occur in a number of disorders such as coeliac disease, ulcerative colitis and Crohn's disease or after prolonged diarrhoea.

The ability to digest lactose is largely inherited and occurs most frequently in adult inhabitants of Northern Europe. Other populations are more likely to experience lactose malabsorption, particularly after childhood, when milk no longer forms such a large part of the diet. About 10% of the adult population in the UK may be intolerance to lactose.

There are wide individual variations in the amount of lactose required to produce symptoms of intolerance. Many lactose-intolerant people can consume about 15 g (the amount contained in half a pint of milk) a day but others can only tolerate much smaller amounts.

As well as being found in milk, lactose is found in yoghurt, ice cream, cream, cheese spreads, soft cheeses such as fromage frais, quark and cottage cheese and spreading fats (particularly very low fat spread). Butter and hard cheeses contain only trace amounts. Foods which are prescribable for lactose intolerance are shown in Table 9.4.

Table 9.4   Products prescribable under ACBS guidelines for lactose intolerance.

Milk formulae
AL110 (Nestlé)
Enfaril Lactafree (Mead Johnson)
Farley's Soya Formula (Farley)
Galactomin Formula 17 (Scientific Hospital Supplies)
InfaSoy (Cow & Gate)
Isomil (Abbott)
Nutramigen (Bristol-Myers)
Pregestimil (Bristol-Myers)
Prejomin (Milupa)
Prosobee (Bristol-Myers)
SMA LF (SMA Nutrition)
Wysoy (Wyeth)
Foods
Comminuted chicken meat (Scientific Hospital Supplies)

Lactose is a common excipient in many medicine formulations, particularly in tablets, and is present in amounts varying from 1 to 500 mg per tablet or capsule. This quantity of lactose is unlikely to cause significant symptoms in many patients but may affect those with severe lactase deficiency. Drug data sheets may give details of lactose content, but for patients who need to avoid lactose for any reason, including veganism, it is better to check with the manufacturer directly.

Glucose and galactose intolerance

Glucose and galactose intolerance cause the same symptoms and are treated in the same way as lactose intolerance, but there is no enzyme deficiency. Lactose is broken down to produce glucose and galactose, but these sugars are not absorbed.

Sucrose intolerance

Sucrose intolerance is much rarer than lactose intolerance and is caused by a deficiency of the enzyme sucrase.

Coeliac disease

Coeliac disease arises from an intolerance to gluten which produces malabsorption of food. About one person in a thousand is affected. Some patients may also be intolerant to lactose. It starts primarily in infancy between the ages of four and six months but is also increasingly diagnosed in adults. The number of infants affected has fallen steadily in recent years, and this may be due to the recommendation that infants under 6 months should not be given foods containing gluten.

Sensitivity to gluten produces intestinal atrophy, but the mechanism by which this occurs is still unknown. Although an immunological reaction may be involved, it is not a simple allergy.

Symptoms include failure to thrive and loss of weight, abdominal distension, flatulence and sometimes vomiting. Impairment in fat absorption leads to fatty diarrhoea which is pale in colour and foul smelling.

Dietary management

The diet must be completely free of gluten. Vitamin and mineral supplementation may be required initially, because malabsorption of food causes nutrient deficiency; this will be prescribed by the doctor.

The prospect of following a gluten-free diet can seem daunting, but a person on a gluten-free diet need not disrupt the rest of the household. If the patient is a child, it is important that everybody involved in the child's care understands the diet. This includes grandparents, aunts and uncles and childminders.

Gluten is found in wheat, rye and barley, and most dietitians also recommend the avoidance of oats. Once the diet has been started, the patient's symptoms improve rapidly. Some common foods which contain gluten, and some which are gluten-free, are shown in Table 9.5.

Table 9.5   Foods classified as containing gluten or gluten-free.

	Gluten-containing foods	Gluten-free-foods
Cereals	Wheat, barley, rye, oats, semolina	Rice, maize, sweetcorn, buckwheat, soya, millet, sago, tapioca, popcorn
	Wheat flour	Arrowroot, cornflour, potato flour, rice flour, soya flour, gluten-free flours
	Wheat and oat bran	Rice and soya bran
	Bread, crispbreads, cakes and biscuits	Gluten-free varieties
	Pasta	Gluten-free pasta
	Breakfast cereals made from wheat, rye, barley or oats	Cornflakes or breakfast cereals made from rice
Raising agents	Baking powders	Bicarbonate of soda, yeast, cream of tartar, gluten-free baking powders and mixes
Meat	Canned meat,[1] meat pastes,[1] pâté,[1] sausages,[1] beefburgers,[1] sausage rolls, pies	Fresh meat, bacon, ham and poultry
Fish	Fish in processed sauces,[1] fish pastes,[1] fish fingers, fishcakes, fish in breadcrumbs or batter	All fresh fish and shellfish
Milk		All milk (fresh, tinned, dried)
Dairy products	Cheese spreads,[1] processed cheese[1]	Plain cheese, cottage cheese, cream cheese, curd cheese, fromage frais
	Synthetic cream,[1] yoghurts[1]	Fresh cream
Spreads and oils	Savoury spreads[1]	Butter, margarine, all cooking oils and fats
Nuts	Peanut butter[1]	Fresh nuts
Seasonings and sauces	Pickles,[1] chutneys,[1] sauces,[1] stock cubes,[1] salad dressings,[1] gravy mixes[1]	Salt, peppercorns, clear vinegar, herbs, pure spices
Soups	Canned and packet soups[1]	Home-made soups with gluten-free ingredients
Fruit	Canned pie fillings[1]	All fresh, canned and frozen fruit
Vegetables	Vegetables canned in sauce[1]	All plain fresh or frozen vegetables
Sweets and jams	Mincemeat,[1] lemon curd,[1] chocolate,[1] sweets,[1] crisps[1]	Sugar, honey, syrup, jam, marmalade
Beverages	Barley flavoured squashes, vending machine drinking chocolate, malted milk drinks	Tea, coffee, most pure fruit juices, pure fruit squashes, fizzy drinks, Complan
Alcohol	Home-made beers	Bought beers, wines and spirits

[1] These foods may or may not contain gluten. Patients should always be referred to the current list of gluten-free foods obtainable from the Coeliac Society and to food manufacturers' labels.

Inadvertent gluten intake is likely to be due to manufactured foods. The most unlikely processed foods (e.g. ice cream and yoghurt) may contain gluten, and different brands of the same types of foods may vary in gluten content. Patients should always be referred to the current list of gluten-free foods which can be obtained from the Coeliac Society, and food labels should always be carefully checked.

Apart from being gluten-free the diet should be as normal as possible, following current healthy eating guidelines (see Chapter 3). Difficulty may arise in ensuring a generous intake of complex carbohydrates because wheat products are a major source in the UK. To help fill this gap there are several proprietary foods, including bread, biscuits, cakes and pasta. Those which are prescribable are shown in Table 9.6, but there are also a number of other products available (mainly cakes and biscuits), which are not prescribable.

Table 9.6   Products prescribable under ACBS guidelines for coeliac disease.

Biscuits, crackers and crispbreads
Aproten (Ultrapharm)
  Biscuits and crispbread
Arnott (Ultrapharm)
  Gluten-free rice cookies
Bi-Aglut (Ultrapharm)
  Biscuits, crackers and cracker toast
Glutafin (Nutricia Dietary)
  Digestive, savoury and sweet biscuits (without chocolate or sultanas), tea
  biscuits, crackers and high fibre crackers
Glutano
  Gluten-free biscuits and crackers
Juvela (Scientific Hospital Supplies)
  Gluten-free digestive, savoury and tea biscuits, and crispbread
Liga (Jacobs)
  Gluten-free rusks
Polial (Ultrapharm)
  Gluten-free biscuits
Schar (Schär)
  Crackers, crispbread, cracker toast, biscuits and savoy biscuits
Ultra (Ultrapharm)
  Crackerbread

Bread
Ener-G (General Dietary)
  Brown rice bread, white rice bread and tapioca bread
Glutafin (Nutricia Dietary)
  Bread and fibre bread and rolls
  Gluten-free bread with soya bran
Juvela (Scientific Hospital Supplies)
  Gluten-free loaf, and bread rolls and high fibre bread rolls
  Low protein, gluten-free loaf (sliced and unsliced)
Lifestyle (Ultrapharm)
  Gluten-free bread rolls, brown bread and white bread

Cont.

Table 9.6 Cont.

Rite-Diet (Nutricia Dietary)
  Gluten-free, white bread and rolls, and high fibre bread and rolls
Schar (Ultrapharm)
  Gluten-free bread, baguette and bread rolls
Sunnyvale (Everfresh)
  Gluten-free bread
Ultra (Ultrapharm)
  Gluten-free baguette, bread, high-fibre bread and rolls
Ultra (Ultrapharm)
  Low protein, gluten-free canned bread (brown and white)
Valpiform (General Dietary)
  Gluten-free loaf

Flour and mixes
Aproten (Ultrapharm)
  Flour
Bar-Kat (Gluten-Free Foods)
  Bread mix
Glutafin (Nutricia Dietary)
  Bread mix and fibre mix
Juvela (Scientific Hospital Supplies)
  Gluten-free harvest mix, bread mix, flour mix
Schar (Schär)
  Gluten-free bread mix, cake mix and pizza base
Tritamyl (Gluten Free Foods Ltd)
  Gluten-free flour, brown bread mix, white bread mix
Trufree (Larkhall)
  Special dietary flours, Nos 1–7
Valpiform (General Dietary)
  Gluten-free bread mix, pastry mix

Pasta and rice
Ener-G (General Dietary)
  Cannelloni, lasagna, shells, small shells, spaghetti, tagliatelle and vermicelli
Glutafin (Nutricia Dietary)
  Spirals, macaroni, and short-cut spaghetti, tagliatelle, vermicelli
Schar (Schär)
  Fusilli, bavette, lasagne, penne, rigatoni, rings, shells, spaghetti and tagliatelle
Tinkyada (General Dietary)
  Brown rice pasta (elbows, fettucini, fusilli, penne, shells, spaghetti, spirals)

Patients should be encouraged to consume generous amounts of gluten-free bread and cereals; otherwise they are likely to choose foods which are high in fat. The taste of different gluten-free breads varies considerably and pharmacists should give advice about different products and encourage patients to try them. For example, gluten-free products which are also low in protein tend to taste less pleasant than those which are just gluten-free.

Several medicines contain gluten, and even the small amount in a tablet may cause problems for a patient with coeliac disease. Some prescribable medicines that contain gluten are shown in Table 9.7, but this does not imply

Table 9.7   Some prescribable medicines which contain gluten.[1]

Apresoline	Navidrex
Lioresal	Rimactazid
Ludiomil	Trasicor (20 and 40 mg only)

[1] This list does not imply that other medicines are gluten-free Individual manufacturers should be contacted.

that all other medicines (particularly generics) are gluten-free. Individual manufacturers should always be contacted.

Inborn errors of metabolism

Causes and symptoms

Inborn errors of metabolism are caused by a genetically determined defect in a single enzyme system, which leads to metabolic disorder. About 200 such disorders are known. The disorder is usually detectable at birth, or soon after, by a clinical or biochemical examination, but sometimes the disorder becomes manifest later in life. Clinical consequences vary considerably; in some the disorder is so severe that the infant may die after a few days or weeks. In others, the disorder may be compatible with a normal lifespan. In those who survive there may be varying degrees of physical and mental disability.

Most of these disorders are extremely rare. Phenylketonuria is the most common, occurring in about 1 in 20 000 births, and is the only inborn error of metabolism which will be discussed in detail. Details of some other inborn errors of metabolism are shown in Table 9.8.

Phenylketonuria

Phenylketonuria (PKU) is a disorder in which there is a deficiency of the enzymes necessary for the breakdown of the amino acid phenylalanine into tyrosine. This causes an increase in the blood level of pehnylalanine, and a decrease in the level of tyrosine. If not detected and treated in early infancy it leads to severe mental retardation. Screening is therefore always carried out after birth.

A diet low in, but not totally excluding, phenylalanine is required; the level of dietary restriction varies from patient to patient. For babies, milk formulas low in phenylalanine must be substituted for breast milk or cow's milk. Extra energy is sometimes required and this can be obtained from carbohydrate or fat supplements.

After weaning, the provision of an adequate diet becomes more complicated, and continuing help from a dietitian is necessary. Some foods such as sugar, jams, sweets and vegetable oils contain negligible amounts of phenylalanine and can be used freely. Fruits and vegetables vary in their

Table 9.8   Inborn errors of metabolism.

Name of disorder	Substance affected	Symptoms	Dietary treatment	Prescribable products
Galactosaemia and galactokinase deficiency	Galactose	Vomiting, feeding difficulties, weight loss, jaundice, cataract, mental and physical retardation	Lactose-free	ALL 110 (Nestlé); Farley's Soya Formula Galactomin Formula 17 (Scientific Hospital Supplies); InfaSoy (Cow & Gate); Isomil (Abbott); Prosobee (Bristol-Myers); Wysoy (Wyeth)
Glucose-6-phosphate dehydrogenase deficiency	Toxins in broad beans	Haemolysis	Avoid broad beans	
Glutaric aciduria	Glutaric acid	Type 1: mental retardation Type 2: multiple metabolic abnormalities	Low lysine, low tryptophan	XLys, Low Try Maxamaid (Scientific Hospital Supplies)
Glycogen storage disease	Glycogen	Growth retardation, enlarged liver, hypoglycaemia, ketoacidosis, occasionally mental retardation	High protein lactose- and sucrose-free	Caloreen (Nestlé Clinical); corn flour; glucose; Maxijul Liquid and Super-Soluble (Scientific Hospital Supplies); Maxijul LE (Scientific Hospital Supplies); Polycal (Nutricia Clinical); Polycose (Abbott); Vitajoule (Vitaflo)
Histidinaemia	Histidine	Delayed development, physical, mental and speech disorders	Low histidine	Various low-protein products
Homocystinuria	Homocysteine, homocystine	Mental retardation, lens dislocation, bone abnormalities	Methionine-free	X Met Analog; Methionine-free Amino Acid mix; XMet Maxamaid; XMet Maxamum (All from Scientific Hospital Supplies)
Hyperlysinaemia	Lysine	Mental retardation	Lysine-free	XLys Analog; XLys Maxamaid (All from Scientific Hospital Supplies)

Cont.

Table 9.8 Cont.

Name of disorder	Substance affected	Symptoms	Dietary treatment	Prescribable products
Hypermethionaemia	Methionine	No specific symptoms, occasional physical and mental handicap	Methionine-free	
Hypoglycaemia	Glucose	Dizziness, mental confusion, sweating	High carbohydrate, low protein, low fat	Caloreen (Nestlé Clinical); corn flour; Maxijul Liquid and Super-Soluble and Maxijul LE (Scientific Hospital Supplies); Polycal (Nutricia Clinical); Polycose (Abbott)
Maple syrup urine disease	Leucine, isoleucine, valine	Feeding difficulties, coma, convulsions, mental retardation	Low in leucine, isoleucine, valine	MSUD Analog; MSUD Maxamaid; MSUD Maxamum; MSUD Aid III (All from Scientific Hospital Supplies)
Methylmalonic or propionic acidaemia	Methylmalonic and propionic acids	Physical and mental retardation	Low in methionine threonine, valine, isoleucine	Methionine, Threonine and Valine-free, Isoleucine-low AA mix; XMet, Thre, Val, Isoleu Analog; XMet, Thre, Val, Isoleu Maxamaid; XMet, Thre, Val, Isoleu Maxamum (All from Scientific Hospital Supplies)
Refsum's disease	Phytanic acid	Peripheral neuropathy, deafness, retinitis	Low in chlorophyll	Fresubin (Fresenius)
Tyrosinaemia	Tyrosine	Type 1: renal damage; Type 2: ocular/skin lesions; psychomotor damage	Low in tyrosine and phenylalanine	XPhen, Tyr Analog; Xphen, Tyr, Met Analog; XPhen, Tyr Maxamaid; Phenylalanine, Tyrosine and Methionine-free Amino Acid mix; Tyrosine and Phenylalanine-free Amino Acid mix (All from Scientific Hospital Supplies)

phenylalanine content; some can be taken freely but others, such as potatoes and Brussels sprouts, can only be used in small quantities. Milk, bread and cereals should also be used with moderation. Bread and cereals should be replaced by low protein alternatives, many of which are available on prescription (see Table 9.9). Foods rich in protein such as meat, fish, cheese and eggs must be avoided. These must be replaced by a protein supplement from which the phenylalanine has been removed.

Table 9.9 Products prescribable under ACBS guidelines for phenylketonuria.

Infant formulae
Lofenalac (Bristol-Myers)

Amino acid supplements
Albumaid XP and XP concentrate (Scientific Hospital Supplies)
Aminogram (UCB Pharma)
LCP Analog (Scientific Hospital Supplies)
XP Analog (for infants from birth to 1 year) (Scientific Hospital Supplies)
Loprofin PKU drink (Scientific Hospital Supplies)
L-Tyrosine (Scientific Hospital Supplies)
XP Maxamaid and XP Maxamaid concentrate (for children of 2–8 years)
    (Scientific Hospital Supplies)
Phlexy-10 Exchange System (Scientific Hospital Supplies)
PK Aid 4 (Scientific Hospital Supplies)
PKU2 and PKU3 (Milupa)

Carbohydrate supplements
Caloreen (Nestlé Clinical)
Polycal (Nutricia Clinical)
Polycose (Abbott)

Fat supplements
Calogen (Scientific Hospital Supplies)

Biscuits, crackers and crispbreads
Aminex (Gluten Free Foods Ltd)
    Low protein biscuits, cookies and rusks
Aproten (Ultrapharm)
    Biscuits and crispbread
dp (Scientific Hospital Supplies)
    Butterscotch-flavoured or chocolate-flavoured chip cookies
Juvela (Scientific Hospital Supplies)
    Low protein, gluten-free chocolate chip, orange or cinnamon-flavoured cookies
Loprofin (Scientific Hospital Supplies)
    Low protein sweet biscuits, chocolate cream filled biscuits, crackers, chocolate
    chip or cinnamon cookies, orange, chocolate or vanilla wafers
Ultra (Ultrapharm)
    PKU biscuits, PKU cookies, PKU savoy biscuits
Valpiform (General Dietary)
    Shortbread biscuits

Bread
Juvela (Scientific Hospital Supplies)
    Low protein, gluten-free loaf (sliced and unsliced), bread rolls

---

Cont.

Table 9.9 Cont.

Loprofin (Scientific Hospital Supplies)
  Low protein bread (sliced and unsliced) and fibre bread (sliced and unsliced)
Ultra (Ultrapharm)
  Low protein, gluten-free canned bread (brown and white)

Flour and mixes
Aproten (Ultrapharm)
  Bread mix, cake mix and flour
Juvela (Scientific Hospital Supplies)
  Low protein, gluten-free flour mix
Rite-Diet (Scientific Hospital Supplies)
  Low protein flour mix and baking mix
Ultra (Ultrapharm)
  PKU flour, pizza base

Pasta and rice
Aglutella (Ultrapharm)
  Low protein rice
Aproten (Ultrapharm)
  Anellini, ditalini, rigatoni, spaghetti and tagliatelle
Loprofin (Scientific Hospital Supplies)
  Macaroni, penne, short-cut spaghetti, spaghetti dough, pasta spirals, vermicelli
Promin (Firstplay Dietary)
  Low protein alphabets, macaroni, shells, shortcut spaghetti, spirals, pasta meal,
  pasta imitation rice

Drinks
Sno-Pro (Scientific Hospital Supplies)

Mineral supplements
Aminogran Mineral Mixture (UCB Pharma)
Metabolic Mineral Mixture (Scientific Hospital Supplies)

Miscellaneous
Loprofin (Scientific Hospital Supplies)
  Egg replacer

Thinking has changed on the diet required for older children and adults. At around 8–10 years of age the brain reaches its maximum capacity. Formerly it was generally considered that the diet could be relaxed. However, it is now though that the patient should remain on the special diet for life. This is particularly important at the time of conception and during pregnancy.

Aspartame is widely used as an artificial sweetener in foods and drinks. It is not suitable for patients with PKU. Aspartame (Canderel) is made in tablet and powder form and it is also added to some soft drinks, fruit juices, flavoured milk drinks, chewing gum, and processed desserts. Food labels should therefore always be checked.

Aspartame is also found in sugar-free medicines, e.g. in granules, powders for antibiotic mixtures, effervescent preparations and chewable tablets. Information about aspartame content may be found in data sheets or on product labels or obtained from manufacturers. If in doubt, sugar-free medicines are best avoided by patients with PKU.

Further reading

National Pharmaceutical Association (1992) Colourants in Oral Liquid Medicines (information leaflet). The National Pharmaceutical Association, St Albans, UK.

Wistow, S. & Bassan, S. (1999) Peanut allergy. *Pharmaceutical Journal*, **262**, 709–710.

Useful addresses

Coeliac Society of the UK, PO Box 220, High Wycombe, Bucks HP11 2HY. Tel: 01494 437278.

Migraine Action Association, 178a High Road, West Byfleet, Surrey KT14 7ED. Tel: 01932 352468.

The Migraine Trust, 45 Great Ormond Street, London WC1N 3HZ. Tel: 0207 278 2676.

National Society for Phenylketonuria and Allied Disorders, 7 Southfield Close, Willen, Milton Keynes, Bucks MK15 9LL. Tel: 01908 691653.

Chapter 10
Anaemias

Anaemia is a reduction in the concentration of haemoglobin below 13 g/100 ml in males or 12 g/100 ml in females. It may be caused by loss of red blood cells, increased destruction or impaired production. Impaired production of red blood cells may be due to deficiency of iron, folic acid or vitamin B_{12}.

Iron deficiency anaemia

Causes

Iron deficiency anaemia may be caused by inadequate iron intake, malabsorption (e.g. coeliac disease) or iron loss due to haemorrhage. Some drugs (e.g. antacids, antibacterials) reduce the absorption of iron.

Susceptible groups of people

Women of child-bearing age are at particular risk because of menstrual losses and pregnancy. The Reference Nutrient Intake (RNI) for such women is 18 mg a day, but many diets do not provide this amount. Iron deficiency is also a risk in infancy and in young people, the elderly, slimmers, athletes, vegetarians, the Asian and Afro-Caribbean communities and people on low incomes.

Prevention

Emphasis should be given to iron-rich foods. Iron is found in a wide variety of both animal and plant foods (see Appendix 3), but with the exception of eggs it is more efficiently absorbed from animal foods. Vitamin C increases the absorption of iron from plant foods, and tannins (contained in tea) reduce it.

Vegetarians should be advised to consume a source of vitamin C at each meal and to drink tea between rather than with meals. Such advice is less important for those who eat meat because absorption of iron from meat is not affected by either vitamin C or tannins.

An iron supplement may be recommended prophylactically for women with heavy menstrual periods or repeated pregnancies. Iron supplements may also be prescribed prophylactically in pregnancy.

Treatment

The oral dose of elemental iron for the treatment of iron deficiency should be between 100 and 200 mg a day (e.g. ferrous sulphate 200 mg three times a day), and the haemoglobin concentration should increase by between 100 and 200 mg/100 ml a day. After the haemoglobin has risen to normal, iron stores should be replenished by continuing the treatment for a further three months. The elemental iron content of iron products is given in Table 10.1.

Table 10.1 Elemental iron content of iron products.

Product	Iron content (mg)
Solid dosage forms (iron content/unit dose)	
Ditemic capsules (SmithKline Beecham)	47 (with vitamins B, C and zinc)
Ferrous fumarate tablets 200 mg	65
Ferrous gluconate tablets 300 mg	35
Ferrous sulphate tablets 200 mg	60
Feospan spansules[1] (Medeva)	47
Ferrograd filmtabs[1] (Abbott)	105
Ferrograd C filmtabs[1] (Abbott)	105 (with vitamin C)
Fersaday tablets (Goldshield)	100
Fersamal tablets (Goldshield)	65
Fesovit Z spansules (Medeva)	47 (with vitamins B, C and zinc)
Galfer capsules (Galen)	100
Givitol capsules (Galen)	100 (with vitamins B & C)
Iron Berries (Seven Seas)	11
Niferex-150 capsules (Tillomed)	150
Slow Fe tablets[1] (Ciba)	50
Liquid dosage forms (iron content/5 ml)	
Ferrous sulphate oral solution	
Paediatric BP	18
Fersamal syrup (Goldshield)	45
Galfer syrup (Galen)	45
Niferex elixir (Tillomed)	100
Plesmet syrup (Link)	25
Sytron elixir (Link)	27.5

[1] Modified-release preparation.

There is little variation in the efficiency of absorption of ferrous salts, but ferric salts are much less well absorbed. Side-effects of iron salts are well known and include constipation or diarrhoea, epigastric pain and nausea. Although modified-release preparations produce fewer side-effects, they may carry the iron to a part of the gut where iron absorption is lower and offer little therapeutic advantage.

Iron interacts with some drugs (e.g. antibacterials, penicillamine) and, if both medicines are necessary, doses should be taken two hours apart.

Megaloblastic anaemia

Causes

Megaloblastic anaemias are caused by deficiency of vitamin B_{12} or folic acid or both. Pernicious anaemia is a particular type of megaloblastic anaemia, in which there is no dietary deficiency but an absence of the gastric intrinsic factor which is essential for the absorption of vitamin B_{12}.

Apart from seaweed, vitamin B_{12} is found naturally only in animal foods. Deficiency may therefore occur in vegans and some vegetarians. Deficiency may occur rarely from the administration of the hypoglycaemic drug metformin, and from excessive alcohol.

Folic acid deficiency may be caused by poor diet, increased physiological demand or malabsorption. It may occur in pregnancy, the elderly and alcoholics or in those taking anti-epileptics such as phenytoin and primidone. The richest food sources of folic acid are liver, yeast products, pulses, wholegrain cereals, green leafy vegetables and nuts.

Treatment

Treatment of megaloblastic anaemia involves identifying the specific deficiency. In an emergency it is sometimes necessary to give both vitamin B_{12} and folic acid while the results of blood tests are being awaited. Folic acid should never be used alone in undiagnosed megaloblastic anaemia because spinal cord degeneration may be precipitated. See Table 10.2 for the iron and folic acid content of some compound products.

Table 10.2   Elemental iron and folic acid content of compound products.

Product	Iron mg	Folic acid μg
Solid oral dose forms (content/unit dose)		
Dencyl capsules (SmithKline Beecham)	47	500 (with vitamins B, C and zinc)
Fefol spansules[1] (Medeva)	47	500
Ferfolic SV tablets[2] (Sinclair)	30	5000 (with vitamin C)
Ferrograd-Folic filmtabs (Abbott)	105	350
Galfer FA capsules (Galen)	100	350
Meterfolic tablets[2] (Sinclair)	100	400
Pregaday tablets (Evans)	100	350
Slow Fe Folic tablets[1] (Ciba)	50	400
Liquid dose form (content/5 ml)		
Lexpec with Iron syrup[2] (Sinclair)	80	2500
Lexpec with Iron-M syrup[2] (Sinclair)	80	500

[1] Modified-release preparation.
[2] Prescription-only medicine (POM).

With the exception of vegans and vegetarians, vitamin B_{12} deficiency is most likely to be caused by malabsorption, so there is no point in giving the vitamin by mouth; hydroxocobalamin injection is given intramuscularly. If the deficiency is caused by diet, cyanocobalamin should be given by mouth.

Chapter 11
Renal Disease

Renal failure leads to impairment in the maintenance of the volume and composition of the body fluids. The aims of management are directed towards maintaining the blood chemistry within normal limits, as well as maintaining any residual kidney function. Treatment involves haemodialysis, haemofiltration, continuous ambulatory peritoneal dialysis (CAPD) or transplantation. Drug dosage may need modification in renal failure (see the British National Formulary).

Dietary management

Dietary modification is usually required and this will be determined by a renal dietitian. Consideration is given to several dietary factors, including protein, energy, sodium, potassium, phosphorus and fluid. The dietary treatment depends on the severity of the disease and also whether the patient is on dialysis. The diet is likely to be much less restrictive once dialysis starts.

Pharmacists may dispense food products for patients with renal failure, and increasingly may help to care for patients who are receiving haemodialysis or CAPD in the community. They should therefore understand the dietary management of renal failure.

Chronic renal failure

Chronic renal failure leads to destruction of the kidney tissue and is an irreversible condition. Hypertension is usually present.

Dietary management

Protein intake is restricted to prevent an excessive rise in blood urea level. An adequate energy intake is essential to ensure that the limited dietary protein and existing body protein in the muscle are not broken down to provide energy. Because protein intake is reduced, most of the required energy must be obtained from carbohydrate and fat.

The sodium content of the diet may need increasing or decreasing depending on the severity of the kidney damage and the ability of the kidneys to excrete sodium. Potassium restriction is usually necessary, and the intake of potassium-rich foods such as coffee, fruit juices, fruit and vegetables must be controlled. Salt substitutes should not be used without medical referral because they have a high potassium content. Phosphorus intake must also be reduced, but protein restriction usually achieves this automatically. Restriction of fluid intake is also important.

Patients with renal disease who have questions about the potassium, sodium and phosphorus content of foods should be referred to their dietitian, because varying amounts are allowed depending on the severity of the disease. Pharmacists should not attempt to give such advice.

Low protein products such as biscuits, bread, flour, pasta and rice are available on prescription (see Table 11.1) and are useful for providing energy and adding variety to the diet. Energy supplements are only needed in patients who are acutely ill or underweight.

Table 11.1   Products prescribable under ACBS guidelines for renal failure.

Biscuits, crackers and crispbreads
Aminex (Gluten Free Foods Ltd)
  Biscuits, cookies and rusks
Aproten (Ultrapharm)
  Biscuits and crispbread
dp (Scientific Hospital Supplies)
  Butterscotch-flavoured or chocolate-flavoured chip cookies
Juvela (Scientific Hospital Supplies)
  Low protein, chocolate chip, orange or cinnamon cookies
Loprofin (Scientific Hospital Supplies)
  Low protein sweet biscuits, chocolate cream-filled biscuits, crackers, chocolate
  chip or cinnamon cookies, orange, chocolate or vanilla wafers
Ultra (Ultrapharm)
  PKU biscuits, PKU cookies, PKU savoy biscuits
Valpiform (General Dietary)
  Low protein shortbread biscuits, cookies with chocolate nuggets

Bread
Juvela (Scientific Hospital Supplies)
  Low protein loaf (sliced and unsliced), bread rolls
Loprofin (Scientific Hospital Supplies)
  Gluten-free, low-protein bread (sliced and unsliced), bread (with or without salt)
Ultra (Ultrapharm)
  Low protein, canned bread (brown and white)

Flour and mixes
Aproten (Ultrapharm)
  Bread mix, cake mix and flour
Juvela (Scientific Hospital Supplies)
  Low protein flour mix
Loprofin (Scientific Hospital Suppliers)
  Low protein, mix
Rite-Diet (Scientific Hospital Supplies)
  Low protein flour mix and baking mix
Ultra (Ultrapharm)
  PKU flour mix, pizza base

Cont.

Table 11.1   Cont.

Pasta and rice
Aglutella (Ultrapharm)
  Low protein rice
Aproten (Ultrapharm)
  Anellini, ditalini, rigatoni, spaghetti and tagliatelle
Loprofin (Scientific Hospital Supplies)
  Macaroni, short-cut spaghetti, pasta spirals, tagliatelle, vermicelli
Promin (Firstplay Dietary)
  Low protein alphabets, macaroni, shells, short-cut spaghetti, spirals, pasta meal,
  pasta imitation rice

Carbohydrate supplements
Caloreen (Nestlé Clinical)
Duocal (Scientific Hospital Supplies)
  Liquid and super-soluble
Hycal (SmithKline Beecham Healthcare)
Maxijul (Scientific Hospital Supplies)
  Liquid and super-soluble
  Maxijul LE
Polycal (Nutricia Clinical)
Polycose (Abbott)

Fat supplements
Calogen (Scientific Hospital Supplies)
Liquigen (Scientific Hospital Supplies)

Amino acid supplement
Dialamine (Scientific Hospital Supplies)

General supplement
Kindergen PROD (Scientific Hospital Supplies)
Nepro (Abbott)
Renamil (Syner-Med)
Suplena (Abbott)

Drinks
Sno-Pro (Scientific Hospital Supplies)

Miscellaneous
Loprofin (Nutricia)
  Egg replacer

Anaemia

Most patients with renal failure have anaemia. This is due mainly to a failure of the damaged kidney to secrete enough erythropoietin to maintain a normal red cell mass. Administration of epoietin (human recombinant erythropoietin) reverses the anaemia completely. Iron and folic acid may also be prescribed.

Renal bone disease

Chronic renal failure results in a disturbance of calcium and phosphate metabolism, with osteomalacia and the risk of aluminium deposition in the bone and brain. These conditions require careful management by a renal specialist.

High plasma phosphate levels can be controlled by diet, and by the use of phosphate-binding agents – either calcium salts or aluminium hydroxide. Calcium salts are now used more widely for phosphate binding than aluminium salts because of the risk of aluminium absorption. Severe hypocalcaemia is treated with vitamin D metabolites (calcitriol and alfacalcidol). Calcium supplements may also be needed.

Acute renal failure

Acute renal failure is commonly caused by circulatory failure due to reduction in blood volume, for example following haemorrhage. It may also occur because of acute nephritis. Urine output falls dramatically, and there is a rapid increase in serum urea and creatinine levels. Hypertension is usually present. Patients often suffer from nausea and vomiting.

Dietary management

The dietary modifications are similar to those used in chronic renal failure, but if the patient is nauseated and has a poor appetite special attention must be paid to energy intake.

Haemodialysis

Haemodialysis involves the removal of water, electrolytes and waste products from the blood using a special apparatus which includes a semipermeable membrane. Most patients undergo dialysis for 4–6 hours, two or three times a week. Haemodialysis is usually carried out in hospital but may also be carried out at home.

Dietary management

The aim of dietary management is to prevent the build-up of fluid, potassium, phosphate and the products of metabolism in between each dialysis session. Protein intake need not be restricted as much for patients who are on dialysis as for those who are not. Some patients who are new to dialysis find it difficult to adjust to this increased protein allowance once haemodialysis has started.

Sodium, potassium and phosphorus restriction is essential. Fluid intake must also be restricted. Energy supplements may be prescribed for patients on haemodialysis (see Table 11.2). Supplementary vitamins and minerals may also be prescribed by the doctor if the patient is on long-term haemodialysis.

Table 11.2   Products prescribable under ACBS guidelines for haemodialysis or continuous ambulatory peritoneal dialysis (CAPD).

Clinitren Dessert (Nestlé Clinical)
Ensure Plus (Abbott)
Formance (Abbott)
Fortipudding (Nutricia Clinical)
Fresubin 750 MCT (Fresenius)
Kindergen PROD[1] (Scientific Hospital Supplies)
Nepro (Abbott)
Protein Forte (Fresenius)
Renapro (Syner-Med)
Suplena (Abbott)

[1] For complete nutritional support or supplementary feeding in children.

Continuous ambulatory peritoneal dialysis

Continuous ambulatory peritoneal dialysis involves the removal of water,
electrolytes and waste products from the blood using the peritoneal membrane as the dialysing membrane. It is now an accepted form of dialysis
treatment, and in the UK more than twice as many patients with end-stage
renal failure are started on CAPD as on haemodialysis. Patients are trained in
hospital to carry out CAPD using aseptic technique so that they can treat
themselves at home. Support for both family and health professionals is very
important for the patient's well being.

Dietary management

In CAPD the removal of products of metabolism is continuous and this
allows a more liberal intake of certain foods. Potassium intake does not
normally need to be restricted, and sodium only needs to be restricted if
blood pressure is high.

Protein is not usually restricted because some is lost during CAPD. Losses
can double during peritonitis which is a risk with this treatment. High
phosphorus intake is discouraged, and, because protein intake is not reduced,
foods high in protein but low in phosphorus should be chosen. Meat and fish
are lower in phosphorus than milk, liver, cheese and eggs.

CAPD may not always be able to provide sufficient dialysis for all patients.
Inadequate dialysis leads to suppression of appetite which can cause
undernourishment. Nutritional status can be improved by using oral supplements (see Table 11.2). Most CAPD patients are given vitamin B and C
supplements to make good losses in the dialysis fluid effluent.

Chapter 12
Liver Disease

Liver disease varies in severity and aetiology, and where dietary management is required this must be supervised by a dietitian. However, pharmacists may dispense food products for chronic liver disease and should understand the reasons for their use.

Liver disease may alter the response to drugs, and their administration should be kept to a minimum in severe liver disease. For a list of drugs to be avoided or used with caution in liver disease, see the British National Formulary.

Chronic liver disease

In chronic liver disease and liver cirrhosis the damaged liver may be unable to metabolise protein, and in these cases a low protein diet is required. There are a number of low protein foods, including biscuits, bread, pasta and rice, which can be prescribed for patients with chronic liver disease and liver cirrhosis (see Table 12.1). Some patients with liver cirrhosis retain sodium and will therefore require a sodium-restricted diet.

Table 12.1 Products prescribable under ACBS guidelines for chronic liver disease.

Biscuits, crackers and crispbreads
Aminex (Gluten Free Foods Ltd)
Biscuits, cookies and rusks
Aproten (Ultrapharm)
Biscuits and crispbread
dp (Scientific Hospital Supplies)
Butterscotch- or chocolate-flavoured chip cookies
Juvela (Scientific Hospital Supplies)
Low protein, chocolate chip, orange- or cinnamon-flavoured cookies
Loprofin (Scientific Hospital Supplies)
Low protein sweet biscuits, chocolate cream filled biscuits, crackers, chocolate chip or cinnamon cookies, orange, chocolate or vanilla wafers
Ultra (Ultrapharm)
PKU biscuits, PKU cookies, PKU savoy biscuits
Valpiform (General Dietary)
Low protein, shortbread biscuits, cookies with chocolate nuggets

Cont.

Table 12.1   Cont.

Bread
Juvela (Scientific Hospital Supplies)
  Low protein loaf (sliced and unsliced), bread rolls
Loprofin (Scientific Hospital Supplies)
  Low protein bread (sliced and unsliced), bread (with or without salt)
Ultra (Ultrapharm)
  Low protein canned bread (brown and white)

Flour and mixes
Aproten (Ultrapharm)
  Bread mix, cake mix and flour
Juvela (Scientific Hospital Supplies)
  Low protein flour mix
Loprofin (Scientific Hospital Supplies)
  Low protein mix
Rite-Diet (Scientific Hospital Supplies)
  Low protein flour mix and baking mix
Ultra (Ultrapharm)
  PKU flour mix, pizza base

Pasta and rice
Aglutella (Ultrapharm)
  Low protein rice
Aproten (Ultrapharm)
  Anellini, ditalini, rigatoni, spaghetti and tagliatelle
Loprofin (Scientific Hospital Supplies)
  Macaroni, short-cut spaghetti, pasta spirals, tagliatelle, vermicelli
Promin (Firstplay Dietary)
  Low protein alphabets, macaroni, shells, short-cut spaghetti, spirals, pasta meal,
  pasta imitation rice

Carbohydrate supplements
Caloreen (Nestlé Clinical)
Duocal (Scientific Hospital Supplies)
  Liquid and super-soluble
Hycal (SmithKline Beecham Healthcare)
Maxijul (Scientific Hospital Supplies)
  Liquid and super-soluble
  Maxijul LE
Polycal (Nutricia Clinical)
Polycose (Abbott)

Fat supplements
Alembicol D (Alembic Products)
Liquigen (Scientific Hospital Supplies)
Medium Chain Triglyceride Oil (Bristol Myers; Scientific Hospital Supplies)

Amino acid supplements
Generaid (Scientific Hospital Supplies)
Generaid Plus (for children over 1 year)
Hepatic Aid (Fresenius)

General supplements
Nepro (Abbott)
Suplena (Abbott)

Miscellaneous
Loprofin (Nutricia)
  Egg replacer

Extra energy may be required and nutritional supplements providing energy in the form of carbohydrate or fat or both, and protein in the form of amino acids are also available on NHS prescription. Additional vitamins and minerals may also be given.

Wilson's disease

Wilson's disease is an inherited disorder which arises out of a failure to store copper by the liver. This leads to excessive deposition of copper in body tissues. It is treated with the drug penicillamine, and pharmacists should be aware that reducing dietary copper intake is impractical and should not be attempted. Penicillamine has the side-effect of chelating zinc, but zinc supplements should not be recommended because penicillamine will preferentially chelate the additional zinc instead of copper, resulting in less copper being removed from the body.

Chapter 13
Musculoskeletal Disorders

Musculoskeletal disorders in which nutrition may be important include osteoporosis, rickets, osteomalacia, arthritis and gout.

Osteoporosis

Osteoporosis is a disorder characterised by a reduction in bone mass, and results in fragile bones, causing fractures. It is predominantly a disease of middle life and old age and affects women more than men.

Risk factors

Bone mass changes throughout life. Peak bone mass is achieved by the third decade with bone loss after the fourth decade. Genetic, hormonal and nutritional factors influence the attainment of peak bone mass, and the onset and rate of bone loss. The decline in oestrogen production after the menopause is associated with bone loss.

Other risk factors include a lower than ideal body weight, particularly a reduced amount of body fat. Asian and Caucasian women appear to be more susceptible than those of Afro-Caribbean origin. Excessive alcohol intake, smoking, inactivity and early menopause are predisposing factors. Diseases such as thyrotoxicosis, hyperparathyroidism and myeloma, and recent corticosteroid therapy, also increase the risk of osteoporosis.

Calcium

The role of calcium in the health of adult bone is a subject of continuing debate, but a growing number of clinical trials show a benefit of supplemental calcium. Vitamin D may also be beneficial either because it improves calcium absorption, or because of a separate and independent effect on bone.

The Reference Nutrient Intake (RNI) for calcium in adult women, including post-menopausal women, is 700 mg a day. The RNI for vitamin D in women over 65 years is 10 µg. There is some evidence that osteoporotic fractures could be reduced by intakes of calcium above this amount: i.e. a daily intake of 1500 mg of calcium for women over the age of 45 years, and particularly for elderly women over the age of 70 years.

A calcium or calcium and vitamin D supplement may be recommended to post-menopausal women, particularly those with one or more risk factors for osteoporosis, but should not be used instead of hormone replacement therapy without medical referral. Appropriate advice should be given abut dose because of the risk of vitamin D toxicity and the fact that excess calcium (> 1 g a day) can cause toxicity in patients with renal failure. Calcium-rich foods should also be emphasised (see Appendix 4).

A calcium supplement should provide 0.5–1 g of elemental calcium per day. Many people are confused by the calcium content of the various calcium supplements available (see Table 13.1). Pharmacists may need to explain that a tablet containing 500 mg of calcium carbonate does not provide 500 mg of calcium.

Table 13.1 Elemental calcium content of some common products.

Supplement	Calcium (mg)
Solid oral dose forms (content/unit dose)	
Calcium gluconate tablets, 600 mg	54
Calcium gluconate effervescent tablets, 1 g	90
Calcium lactate tablets, 300 mg	40
Calcium and ergocalciferol tablets	
(calcium and vitamin D)	97 (with 10 µg vitamin D)
Cacit D3 (Procter & Gamble)	500 (with 11 µg vitamin D)
Cacit tablets (Procter & Gamble)	500
Calceos (Thames)	500 (with 10 µg vitamin D)
Calcia tablets (English Grains)	250
Calcichew tablets (Shire)	500
Calcichew-D3 tablets (Shire)	500 (with 5 µg vitamin D)
Calcichew D3 Forte (Shire)	500 (with 10 µg vitamin D)
Calcichew Forte tablets (Shire)	1000
Calcidrink granules (Shire)	1000
Calcium-500 tablets (Martindale)	500
Ostram powder (Merck)	1200
Sandocal-400 tablets (Novartis)	400
Sandocal-1000 tablets (Novartis)	1000
Seven Seas calcium berries (Seven Seas)	500 (with 6.25 µg vitamin D)
Liquid dose form (content/5 ml)	
Calcium-Sandoz syrup (Alliance)	108

One of the best protections against osteoporosis is to enter middle life with a high bone density. This can be achieved by stressing the importance of calcium-rich foods before the tike when peak bone mass is achieved. This usually occurs at about 30–35 years of age. Skeletal growth is particularly rapid during the teenage years, and the importance of calcium should therefore be emphasised in the diet of young people.

Advice for reducing the risk of osteoporosis is summarised below:

> **Advice to help reduce the risk of osteoporosis.**
>
> (1) Emphasise calcium-rich foods in the diet (see Appendix 4)
> (2) Exercise three times a week (preferably weight-bearing exercise such as jogging, walking and racquet sports)
> (3) Reduce alcohol consumption
> (4) Stop smoking

Rickets and osteomalacia

Rickets is a disease of children and is characterised by impairment of mineralisation in which the bones are softened and deformed. Osteomalacia is the adult counterpart of rickets.

Causes

Both rickets and osteomalacia arise as a result of vitamin D deficiency, which leads to a failure to absorb calcium. Vitamin D is synthesised in the skin during exposure to sunlight and is also obtained from the diet. There are few dietary sources of vitamin D (see Appendix 5), but cutaneous synthesis is normally efficient.

Vitamin D deficiency occurs when supply from both sources is defective, or there is an increased requirement. Gastrointestinal surgery or coeliac disease may lead to malabsorption. Disorders of parathyroid function and chronic renal and liver disease may lead to defective metabolism of the vitamin. Prolonged use of anticonvulsants can also cause vitamin D deficiency.

At risk groups

Groups of people at risk of developing rickets and osteomalacia include

- Children from low-income households
- Elderly people
- Asians, particularly during infancy, childhood, adolescence and pregnancy
- Patients with malabsorption conditions, chronic liver disease and renal disease
- Patients on long-term anticonvulsant therapy

Prevention

Prevention is best achieved by providing vitamin D supplements (10 µg or 400 IU/day) for groups of people at risk of developing rickets and osteomalacia, particularly infants and children from the age of 6 months to 5 years, pregnant women and the elderly. The consumption of vitamin D-rich foods (see Appendix 5), including foods fortified with the vitamin (e.g. breakfast cereals), should also be encouraged.

Exposure to sunlight is important, but because of the northerly latitude of the UK, ultraviolet light of the wavelength required for vitamin D synthesis only reaches northern parts of the UK between May and September. However, even short periods of summer sunlight (15–30 minutes a day) with exposure of face, hands and forearms will lead to production of adequate amounts.

Treatment

Rickets and osteomalacia are treated with vitamin D, and supplemental calcium may also be given to promoted remineralisation of the skeleton. In simple nutritional rickets and osteomalacia, the dose of vitamin D varies from 25 to 100 μg (1000 to 4000 IU)/day depending on the severity of the disease.

In patients with malabsorption, or chronic liver or renal disease, vitamin D is usually required in pharmacological doses of up to 2.5 mg (100 000 IU)/ day or more. Once major deformities are present they can only be corrected by orthopaedic surgery.

Arthritis

There are several types of arthritis but rheumatoid arthritis and osteoarthritis are the most common. As yet there is no cure for arthritic conditions, and treatment involves drugs, physiotherapy and surgery.

Diet

The use of particular diets in arthritis is controversial, and pharmacists may be asked about them. Many patients alter their diets and claim relief from their symptoms, but arthritis naturally tends to go through phases of improvement and relapse so any improvement could be coincidental.

Claims have been made that arthritis is linked to food allergy, and certain foods may exacerbate the symptoms in some people. If food allergy is suspected, the patient should be referred to a dietitian, who may try excluding the food or foods in question. Patients should be discouraged from self-diagnosis and self-treatment of suspected food allergies, because the diet may become too restrictive increasing the risk of nutrient deficiency.

While there is little evidence for the benefit of special diets in arthritis, obesity increases the load on the muscles and joints. Patients with arthritis should be advised to eat a healthy diet and lose weight if appropriate.

Dietary supplements

Both fish oils and fish liver oils are now commonly taken for arthritis, and many patients claim relief from their symptoms. It is the n-3 polyunsaturated fatty acids in these oils which may be beneficial in arthritis because they affect prostaglandin production. Prostaglandins influence the inflammatory process.

Some books and magazine articles advise dangerously large doses of these oils, and pharmacists should warn people taking fish liver oils about the dangers of vitamin A and D toxicity. This is not a problem with fish oil (as opposed to fish liver oil) supplements, because they contain much smaller amounts of these vitamins.

Pharmacists are often asked about the difference between the fish liver oil and the capsules. While the recommended dose of oil generally provides the same amounts of vitamins A and D as the recommended dose of capsules, the oil generally provides more of the n-3 polyunsaturated fatty acids (see Table 25.4.

Large doses of vitamin C have also been claimed to benefit arthritis but there is little scientific evidence for this.

Gout

Gout is caused by the deposition of urate crystals in the joints and is associated with an increased concentration of urate in the plasma. It is a disease of affluence, and it was recognised in the eighteenth century that large meals and alcohol often precipitated an attack. Raised urate level is a result of excessive production, or decreased renal excretion of uric acid, or both. Only a small part of the excess uric acid is caused by dietary purines.

Gout is treated with drugs. Non-steroidal anti inflammatory drugs (NSAIDs) and colchicine are used in acute attacks, and allopurinal and other uricosuric drugs are used in the long-term control of the disease.

Diet

Uricosuric drugs are generally effective in controlling gout, and a strict low purine diet is not necessary. However, rich sources of purines should be avoided. These include offal, such as liver, heart, kidney and sweetbreads, fish such as anchovies, sardines, herring and mackerel, seafood such as shrimps and crab, fish roes and meat extracts.

Overweight patients should be advised to lose weight but they should achieve this gradually. Fasting or strict dieting increases blood uric acid levels and is likely to do more harm than good.

Because there is a risk of renal stones in gout, patients should be advised to drink at least 8 cups of fluid every day. Coffee, tea, water and fruit juices may be consumed, but alcohol should be restricted to 1 unit a day. This means no more than one glass of wine or half a pint of beer. For more explanation of alcohol units, see Chapter 3.

The diet should be based on healthy eating principles. Too much food and alcohol should be avoided because this may precipitate an attack of gout.

Useful addresses

Arthritic Association, Hill House, 1 Little New Street, London EC4A 3TR. Tel: 0207 491 0233.

Arthritis Care, 18 Stephenson Way, London NW1 2HD. Tel: 0207 916 1500 or 0800 289170.

National Osteoporosis Society, PO Box 10, Radstock, Bath, BA3 3YB. Tel: 01761 471771.

Chapter 14
Skin

This chapter will consider the role of diet in some skin diseases which commonly present in pharmacies and for which patients may believe there is some dietary treatment. These include eczema, psoriasis and acne. Dermatitis herpetiformis will also be discussed.

Eczema and psoriasis

There is no justification for dietary modifications in eczema and psoriasis.

Vitamin A has been claimed to be of value, but in physiological doses it is unlikely to produce any benefit. At 200 times the physiological dose vitamin A may exert an antiproliferative effect in skin which is a pharmacological response. Synthetic vitamin A derivatives (retinoids) produce a more beneficial therapeutic response and are used in the treatment of eczema and psoriasis. They are extremely toxic, so careful monitoring is necessary.

Evening primrose oil is claimed to be of benefit in the symptomatic relief of eczema, and is available as a dietary supplement and as a prescribable medicine.

Acne

Acne, a common disorder in teenagers, is often associated with eating chocolate and fatty foods. There is little evidence to support this view, but these foods should in any case be eaten in moderation.

Synthetic vitamin A derivatives (retinoids) are used to treat acne (see above).

Dermatitis herpetiformis

Dermatitis herpetiformis is a chronic skin disorder which is frequently associated with coeliac disease. It is characterised by intense itching and blistering on the buttocks, knees, elbows and shoulders.

Most patients with this skin disorder are sensitive to gluten and benefit greatly from a gluten-free diet (see Chapter 9) although it may take several months for the skin lesions to clear up. Foods which are prescribable for coeliac disease (see Table 9.6) are also prescribable for dermatitis herpetiformis.

Useful addresses

National Eczema Society, 163 Eversholt Street, London NW1 1BU. Tel: 0207 388 4097.

Section 4
Diet throughout the Life Cycle

Chapter 15
Pregnancy and Lactation

Everybody should be advised to eat a healthy diet, but this is particularly important during pregnancy and lactation because of the influence of nutrition on the infant's health. Although dietary guidelines for pregnancy and lactation do not differ significantly from those for other healthy adults, women tend to be particularly receptive to nutritional advice at this time. Like other health professionals, pharmacists should make the most of this opportunity to encourage healthy eating.

Before conception

Dietary advice before conception is particularly important because one of the most significant influences on the infant's birthweight is the mother's nutritional state at the start of pregnancy. Requests for ovulation kits and pregnancy tests may provide pharmacists with opportunities for encouraging healthy eating.

Body weight

Ideal weight should be attained before pregnancy starts. Being overweight increases the chance of the mother having too heavy a baby, and also of gestational diabetes and hypertension.

Nutrients

It is important that the body's stores of all nutrients are optimal before conception. This can be achieved by eating a varied diet based on the healthy eating guidelines (see Chapter 3).

Folic acid

Folic acid is an essential nutrient throughout pregnancy, but is particularly important in early pregnancy. An inadequate intake of folate before the time of neural tube closure (about 28 days after conception) increases the risk of neural tube defects (e.g. spina bifida and anencephalopathy). Folic acid supplementation has been shown to reduce the risk of neural tube defect occurrence.

The Department of Health now recommends that all women who are planning a pregnancy, or who may become pregnant, should take a folic acid supplement. Supplementation should continue until the 12th week of pregnancy. Different doses are recommended depending on the level of risk (see Table 15.1). In addition, women should be advised to increase their intake of folate-rich foods (see Table 15.2).

Anti-epileptic drugs, such as phenytoin, interfere with folate metabolism so women taking these drugs who are planning a pregnancy should be referred to the doctor.

Table 15.1 Doses of folic acid before conception and during pregnancy.

	Dose
High risk[1]	5 mg daily
Low risk[2]	0.4 mg daily

[1] Women judged to be at high risk of producing an infant with a neural tube defect.
[2] Women judged to be at low risk of producing an infant with a neural tube defect.

Table 15.2 Dietary sources of folate.

Food	Folate content (µg)
2 slices lamb's liver[1]	250
1 cup Bovril	95
Yeast spread on 1 slice of bread	40
Milk (1 pint)	35
2 slices white bread	16
2 slices wholemeal bread	30
2 slices fortified bread (fortified with folic acid)	60
1 bowl cornflakes (unfortified)	3
1 bowl cornflakes (fortified)	100
1 bowl bran flakes (unfortified)	40
1 bowl bran flakes (fortified)	100
1 bowl muesli	60
1 serving Brussels sprouts	100
1 serving spinach	80
1 serving green beans	50
1 serving potatoes	45
1 serving cauliflower	45
1 serving baked beans	50
1 orange	50
1 glass orange juice	40

[1] Pregnant women and those planning a pregnancy are advised to avoid liver or liver products.

Vitamin A

An adequate intake of vitamin A is required before conception, but excessive amounts can substantially increase the risk of birth defects. The Department of Health has warned women who could become pregnant to avoid eating liver and liver products such as liver sausage and pâté. This is because liver is a particularly concentrated source of vitamin A.

Women planning a pregnancy should also be advised to avoid dietary supplements containing large amounts of Vitamin A (in the form of retinol). This recommendation has caused some confusion. It does not mean that vitamin A should be avoided altogether – in any case it would be difficult to eat a diet devoid of vitamin A – but most women consume more vitamin A than they require in the diet. Thus, to avoid excessive intake, dietary supplements containing vitamin A in excess of the RDA should be avoided. Supplements containing vitamin A in the form of beta-carotene are safe, because beta-carotene, a precursor of vitamin A, is converted to vitamin A only in amounts that the body needs.

Alcohol

Alcohol can affect the absorption and metabolism of a number of nutrients, particularly trace minerals, and is best avoided or at least restricted to a couple of glasses of wine or the equivalent each week.

Oral contraceptives

Oral contraceptives may prejudice trace mineral and vitamin status, although this risk is probably less now than before when the oestrogen content of the pill was higher. Nevertheless, it is a wise precaution to stop taking oral contraceptives three months before conception is planned.

Nutritional advice for women planning a pregnancy.

(1) Eat a diet based on healthy eating guidelines
(2) Increase intake of folate-rich foods
(3) Take a supplement of folic acid until the 12th week of pregnancy (see Table 15.1)
(4) Avoid liver or products containing it
(5) Avoid dietary supplements containing excessive vitamin A
(6) Avoid or restrict alcohol intake
(7) Stop taking oral contraceptives 3 months before planned conception

---

Pregnancy

Pregnancy and the needs of the growing foetus impose increased nutritional demands on the mother, but large increases in nutrient intake are not required. This is partly because absorption of many nutrients increases, excretion decreases and metabolism is generally more efficient.

Energy and nutrients

The extra energy and nutrients required during pregnancy are shown in Table 15.3; for absolute requirements see Appendix 1. Requirements for nutrients can generally be met by eating a varied and healthy diet. If the mother's diet is inadequate, the infant will take whatever it requires from the maternal stores. This will result in nutrient deficiency in the mother, particularly if her nutrient stores are low.

Table 15.3 Additional daily energy[1] and nutrient[2] requirements for pregnancy and lactation.

	Pregnancy	Lactation
Energy (MJ/kcal)	0.8 (200)[3]	1.90 (450 at 1 month
		2.20 (530) at 2 months
		2.40 (570) at 3 months
		2.00 (480) at 4–6 months[4]
		2.40 (570) at 4–6 months[5]
		1.00 (240) at > 6 months[4]
		2.30 (550) at > 6 months[5]
Protein (g)	6	11 at 0–4 months
		8 at > 4 months
Thiamin (mg)	0.1	0.2
Riboflavin (mg)	0.3	0.5
Niacin (mg)	*	2.0
Vitamin B_6 (mg)	*	*
Vitamin B_{12} (µg)	*	0.5
Folate (µg)	6	60
Vitamin C (mg)	10	30
Vitamin A (µg)	100	350
Vitamin D (µg)	10	10
Calcium (mg)	*	550
Phosphorus (mg)	*	440
Magnesium (mg)	50	50
Sodium (mg)	*	*
Potassium (mg)	*	*
Iron (mg)	*	*
Zinc (mg)	*	6 at 0–4 months
		2.5 >4 months
Copper (mg)	*	0.3
Selenium (µg)	*	15
Iodine (µg)	*	*

* No increment.
[1] Estimated average requirement (EAR).
[2] Reference Nutrient Intake (RNI).
[3] Last trimester only.
[4] For women who wean the infant over a period of a few months.
[5] For women whose intention is that breast milk should provide the primary source of nourishment for 6 months or more.
[6] See Table 15.1.

Energy

An adequate energy intake is essential during pregnancy, both for the growth and development of the foetus and also for the development of the mother's stores of adipose tissue for lactation. However, it is neither necessary nor desirable to 'eat for two'; the DOH has recommended an average increase in energy intake of 0.8 MJ (200 kcal), and that only in the last trimester. Excessive energy intake will obviously lead to undesirable weight gain, and this may result in the production of too heavy an infant as well as hypertension in the mother. On the other hand, if energy intake is inadequate, the risk of a low birthweight infant increases, particularly in underweight women. Women should therefore always be discouraged from attempting to slim during pregnancy. Ideal weight should, if possible, be attained before conception.

Probably the best guideline for energy intake is the achievement of desirable weight gain in the mother. This varies depending on her initial weight as follows:

- 9 kg for women who are in the ideal weight range (i.e. between 80 and 120% of ideal body weight) at the start of pregnancy
- 13.5 kg for women who are underweight (i.e. less than 80% of ideal weight) at the start of pregnancy
- 7.5 kg for women who are overweight (i.e. more than 120% of ideal weight) at the start of pregnancy

Provided weight gain falls within desirable limits, there is no need to worry about energy intake. Women normally gain about 4 kg by the end of the 20th week and then about 0.5 kg/week until term.

Iron

The need for supplemental iron during pregnancy has been debated extensively. Haemoglobin values do fall during pregnancy but this is a natural consequence of the increase in blood volume; it does not necessarily mean that the woman is anaemic. Iron losses are in any case reduced because menstruation ceases.

Currently, it is generally agreed that foetal iron requirement can be met from maternal stores without the mother taking any extra iron. The DOH recommends no increment in iron intake above that for the average adult woman. This does not mean that iron requirements should be ignored during pregnancy. Women should be advised to eat iron-rich foods (see Appendix 3). For vegetarian women it is particularly important to eat foods rich in vitamin C. This is because iron from vegetarian sources is less well absorbed than iron from animal sources. Iron absorption from plant foods is increased by consuming vitamin C-rich foods at the same meal. A small glass of orange juice, a citrus fruit, salad or a green vegetable at every meal will maximise iron absorption.

Iron supplements are required by women who have low iron stores at the start of pregnancy. Because there is no cheap and quick method for measuring iron stores, many women continue to be prescribed iron supplements without knowing whether they need them or not. Women likely to have poor iron status are those who have heavy periods and those who have had several pregnancies in close succession. Some vegetarian women and those on low incomes may also suffer from iron deficiency.

Folic acid

Folic acid has traditionally been prescribed during pregnancy to prevent megaloblastic anaemia, but there is now evidence that folic acid also has a role in the prevention of neural tube defects.

The DOH recommends that supplements should be taken by all pregnant women, starting from the time when they begin planning a pregnancy until at least the 12th week of pregnancy. If an unplanned pregnancy occurs, folic acid supplementation should start immediately. Recommended doses of folic acid are different depending on the level of risk of producing an affected infant (see Table 15.5). All pregnant women should be advised to increase their intake of folate-rich foods (see Table 15.2). Supplements containing 400 μg of folic acid are available from the following manufacturers: English Grains (Folic Plus), Health & Diet Food (FSC), Health Plus, Lambert's, Lane's (Preconceive), Larkhall, Nature's Best, Pharmadass (Health Aid) and Solgar.

Calcium

Extra calcium is required by the foetus, but absorption of dietary calcium increases during pregnancy and doubles by the 24th week. Although no increment is recommended for calcium intake during pregnancy, women should be encouraged to each calcium-rich foods (see Appendix 4). Vegan women often have low intakes and may require a supplement.

Vitamin A

An adequate intake of vitamin A is required during pregnancy but excessive intakes are associated with an increased risk of birth defects. The DOH recommends that foods particularly rich in vitamin A such as liver and liver products be avoided during pregnancy as well as in women planning a pregnancy. Dietary supplements containing vitamin A in amounts exceeding RDA should also be avoided. These recommendations have led to some confusion and women may believe that they should avoid vitamin A entirely. This is not true; it is just excessive intakes that should be avoided.

Vitamin D

Vitamin D requirements are largely obtained by the action of sunlight on the skin, and for most women dietary vitamin D is less important. Vitamin D deficiency is common in mothers and infants especially during the winter and early spring in areas where sunlight is scarce. Attention should therefore be given to improving dietary vitamin D intake during pregnancy, and a daily intake of 10 µg is recommended. Few diets regularly contain this amount, so pregnant women should be encouraged to eat foods which contain vitamin D (see Appendix 5) and possibly to take a supplement.

Asian and vegan women are at particular risk of vitamin D deficiency, partly because they are unlikely to be eating the foods which contain it. A supplement is therefore a wise precaution.

Vitamin B_{12}

An omnivorous diet will easily provide the requirement for vitamin B_{12} during pregnancy but a vegan diet will be lacking in the vitamin. Pregnant women who are vegans will need to take a supplement.

Dietary advice for common problems

Nausea and vomiting

Nausea and vomiting are common, particularly in early pregnancy, but usually subside by the 16th week. Occasionally women suffer throughout pregnancy. Provided that weight gain falls within the desirable range, it is unlikely that sickness will harm the foetus. These symptoms cause great discomfort to the prospective mother who may benefit from eating frequent snacks and smaller meals. There is no harm in snacks replacing full meals provided that the snacks are nutritious. Suitable snacks include:

- Plain biscuits or crackers
- Bread or toast, either plain or with yeast spread or cottage cheese
- Soup
- Breakfast cereals
- Sandwiches
- Hot or cold milk drinks
- Yoghurt
- Fresh fruit or raw vegetables
- Jacket potato

Heartburn and indigestion

These are common problems during pregnancy as the growing womb starts to press on the stomach. The following advice may be helpful:

- Avoiding any foods which cause the symptoms
- Eating smaller meals more frequently

- Eating slowly
- Avoiding heavy meals near bedtime

An antacid may be prescribed, but pharmacists should remember that, if an iron supplement is being taken, the two preparations should be administered at least 2 hours apart. This is because antacids can reduce the absorption of iron.

Constipation

Gastrointestinal motility slows in pregnancy, probably because of hormonal changes, and constipation may be a problem. Women should be advised to increase their intake of non-starch polysaccharides (NSP) by eating wholemeal bread, brown pasta and rice, wholegrain cereals, pulses, and fruit and vegetables. Fluid intake should be increased at the same time.

Cravings

Cravings and taste alterations are common in pregnancy. Provided that the diet is not substantially altered, there is no danger to either the mother or infant. Many women just 'go off' tea or coffee, which is not harmful, but cravings for sweet, fatty foods may encourage excessive weight gain and reduce the appetite for more nutritious foods.

Listeria

Listeria has received a great deal of publicity. Although a rare disease, it can be dangerous if it occurs in pregnancy and may lead to miscarriage, stillbirths and septicaemia in the infant. Early symptoms are often flu-like, and any pregnant woman with such symptoms should be referred to the doctor immediately.

Some cases of listeria have been associated with food, and strict food hygiene practices should be emphasised (see Chapter 4). In addition the following foods should be avoided:

- undercooked poultry or meat products
- any kind of pâté
- salads, raw vegetables and fruit which is unwashed
- soft mould-ripened cheese such as Brie, Camembert and blue-veined varieties. Hard cheeses such as Cheshire and Cheddar are safe. Cream cheese, cottage cheese and fromage frais are also safe provided they are processed.

Nutritional advice during pregnancy.

(1) Eat a varied diet based on healthy eating guidelines
(2) Avoid or restrict the intake of alcohol
(3) Emphasise folate-rich foods
(4) Take folate supplements[1] until at least the 12th week
(5) Emphasise iron- and calcium-rich foods
(6) Avoid liver and liver products
(7) Avoid dietary supplements containing excessive vitamin A

[1] See Table 15.1

Lactation

The purpose of this section is to discuss the nutritional needs of the mother during lactation (see the box at the end of this section). The nutritional value of breast milk to the infant will be discussed in Chapter 16.

Energy and nutrients

The extra amounts of energy and nutrients required for lactation have been specified by the DOH (1991) and are summarised in Table 15.3.

Energy

The amount of energy required to produce breast milk is large, and varies between 1.9 MJ (450 kcal) a day when the infant is 1 month old to 2.4 MJ (570 kcal) a day when the infant is 4 months old. This extra energy can easily be provided by the mother's diet which should be based on healthy eating guidelines.

Vitamins and minerals

Some vitamins and minerals are required in increased amounts (see Table 15.3), and such requirements can normally be met from the increased energy intake provided the diet is varied and healthy. The requirement for calcium nearly doubles during lactation, so special attention should be given to foods rich in calcium (see Appendix 4).

Dietary supplements

Most mothers do not need dietary supplements but vegans should take a supplement containing vitamin B_{12}, vitamin D and calcium. Asian mothers may be at risk of vitamin D deficiency which could be passed on to the infant, and they may need a vitamin D supplement. Pharmacists should remember the possibility of overdosage with vitamin D and advise the mother accordingly. Excessive doses of vitamin D in the mother could lead to hypercalcaemia in the infant.

Fluid

Fluid is essential for establishing and maintaining lactation. Mothers should therefore be advised to drink whenever they feel thirsty, bearing in mind, though, that large quantities of tea, coffee and cola drinks are best avoided since excess caffeine might prevent the infant from sleeping. Alcohol should be avoided or restricted to no more than one or two glasses of wine a week.

Nutritional advice during lactation.

(1) Eat a varied diet based on healthy eating guidelines
(2) Eat according to appetite; do not be afraid to eat more if hungry
(3) Emphasise foods rich in calcium
(4) Drink plenty of fluid
(5) Restrict the intake of alcohol, tea, coffee and cola drinks

---

Further reading

DOH (1991) Dietary reference values for food energy and nutrients for the United Kingdom. Report on Health and Social Subjects No 41, HMSO, London.

DOH (1992) Folic Acid and the Prevention of Neural Tube Defects. Report from an Expert Advisory Group. Available from Health Publications Unit, Heywood Stores, No 2 Site, Manchester Road, Heywood, Lancashire OL10 2PZ.

Useful addresses

Association of Breastfeeding Mothers, PO Box 441, St Albans, Hertfordshire AL4 0AS. Tel: 01727 859189.

La Lèche League of Great Britain, BM3424, London WC1N 3XX. Tel: 0207 242 1278.

Maternity Alliance, 45 Beech Street, London EC2P 2LX.

National Childbirth Trust, Alexandra House, Oldham Terrace, Acton, London W3 6NH. Tel: 0208 992 8637.

Women's Nutritional Advisory Service, PO Box 268, Lewes, East Sussex BN7 2QN. Tel: 01273 487366.

Chapter 16
Infants

Good nutrition is important in infancy not only to promote growth and development but also because it may contribute to disease prevention in adult life. The risk of developing obesity, hypertension, coronary heart disease, diabetes mellitus and cancer may be altered by diet in the first few weeks and months of life. Because parents of infants are such frequent visitors to community pharmacies, pharmacists can make an important contribution to the health and well-being of future generations.

This chapter will discuss the nutritional needs and advice which can be given to parents and carers of infants up to the age of 1 year. Dietary advice for older children and adolescents is discussed in Chapter 17.

Choice of feeding method

Milk provides all the nutrients required by the growing infant during the first few months of life, and a significant proportion of nutrients thereafter. Deciding whether to breast or bottle feed can be difficult, and is likely to be influenced by the mother's background and environment, including her attitudes, experiences and beliefs and those of her mother, partner and friends.

The provision of information to help parents make a choice is vital. Women in higher social classes are likely to read books and leaflets on the subject, but women in lower social classes may need special attention. Pharmacists can provide such information but should not attempt to make up mothers' minds for them. After the birth, mothers should be supported in whichever method they have chosen, and their choice should be respected.

Breast feeding

Breast milk is considered to be the best source of nutrition for the new-born infant and for at least the first six months of life. It may be continued as part of mixed feeding until the baby is 12 months old, and some mothers choose to carry on for longer.

The incidence of breast feeding in the UK increased during the period 1975 to 1980 but there has been little change since. About 65% of mothers breast feed their infants at birth but this figure falls to about 40% by the end of the 6th week and about 20% by 6 months.

Breast feeding is more common in women from the higher social classes, those over 25 years of age, those living in the South-East of England and those who have been educated beyond the age of 18. First and second babies are more commonly breast fed than babies born later in the family.

The advantages and disadvantages of breast feeding

Advantages

(1) Breast milk provides the perfect balance of energy and nutrients for healthy growth and development.

(2) Some nutrients such as iron, zinc, calcium and fat are better absorbed from breast milk.

(3) The concentration of solutes in breast milk is regulated naturally; there is no risk of solute overload.

(4) Breast milk needs no preparation.

(5) Breast milk provides protection against infection, both bacterial and viral. It contains antibodies to bacteria such as *Haemophilus influenzae*, *Klebsiella*, *Salmonella* and *Streptococcus pneumoniae*. It also contains immunoglobulins (especially IgA), bifidus factor, lactoferrin, lymphocytes, lysozyme and macrophages. IgA may help to prevent food allergy and atopic eczema.

(6) Breast milk may have a beneficial effect on neuro-development. Recent research suggests that breast milk may improve intelligence, but further work is needed to confirm this.

(7) Breast feeding may help to prevent obesity, cardiovascular disease, cancer and diabetes mellitus in later life.

(8) Breast feeding helps maternal bonding. This is important for the emotional and physical development of the child.

(9) Breast feeding is relatively cheap even considering the extra nutritional needs of the lactating mother.

(10) Breast feeding has benefits for the mother. It helps the uterus to return to its original size and shape and also helps to utilise surplus body fat deposited in pregnancy.

(11) Breast feeding has a mile contraceptive effect but parents should be warned that this is not an efficient method of contraception.

Disadvantages

(1) Breast feeding is tying for the mother; she must be available day and night, particularly during the early weeks.

(2)   It can create jealousy in husbands, partners and other children in the family.

(3)   Mothers may worry because they cannot see the volume of milk being taken, but any infant who is contented and gaining weight is adequately fed.

(4)   There may be problems in establishing and maintaining lactation or the milk supply may be inadequate.

(5)   Full breast feeding is likely to be impossible of the mother returns to work, but partial breast feeding can usually be continued and should be encouraged.

(6)   Drugs may be transferred to the infant in the breast milk. For a list of drugs to be avoided during breast feeding, see the British National Formulary.

(7)   Human milk is unsuitable for infants with some inherited disorders of metabolism (e.g. galactosaemia and phenylketonuria).

The composition of breast milk

The composition of breast milk changes during the days after the birth. Immediately after birth the secretion is a thick, yellow milk called colostrum. Colostrum is higher in protein, vitamin A, vitamin E and vitamin B_{12} than mature breast milk but lower in fat content. It supplies all the nutrients required by the baby during the first few days of life. Colostrum also supplies a high concentration of antibodies, which limits the multiplication of bacteria and viruses in the gastrointestinal tract.

After 3 to 4 days the milk becomes thinner and whiter and approaches the composition of mature milk, which begins to be produced between the seventh and tenth days after birth. The composition and volume vary among mothers, and the volume also depends on the demands of the infant.

Milk composition changes during the course of a feed. Fat and energy content of the milk is higher at the end than the beginning of the feed. If a feed is ended too rapidly, the baby will be deprived of the most energy-dense part with a consequent failure to thrive.

The mean composition of mature breast milk is shown in Table 16.1. The proportion of energy provided by fat is high compared with dietary guidelines for adults, and the protein content is lower. About two-thirds of the protein is in the form of whey which is more easily digested than casein. Carbohydrate is provided in the form of lactose.

The vitamin, mineral and trace element content of breast milk should be adequate to supply all the infant's needs unless the mother's diet is deficient.

Establishing and maintaining breast feeding

The infant should be put to the breast immediately after delivery in order to develop the suckling reflex. Thereafter the baby should be fed about every 2–

Table 16.1   Mean composition of mature breast milk.

Energy (kJ)	293
(kcal)	70
Protein (g)	1.3
Fat (g)	4.1
Carbohydrate (g)	7.2
Vitamin A (µg)	60
Thiamin (mg)	0.02
Riboflavin (mg)	0.03
Niacin (mg)	0.22
Vitamin B_6 (mg)	0.01
Vitamin B_{12} (µg)	0.01
Folate (µg)	5
Pantothenic acid (mg)	0.3
Biotin (µg)	0.7
Vitamin C (mg)	4
Vitamin D (µg)	0.04
Vitamin E (mg)	0.3
Vitamin K (µg)	0.3
Calcium (mg)	34
Phosphorus (mg)	15
Magnesium (mg)	2.8
Sodium (mg)	15
Potassium (mg)	60
Chloride (mg)	45
Iron (mg)	0.07
Zinc (mg)	0.3
Copper (mg)	0.04
Selenium (µg)	1.4
Iodine (µg)	7
Manganese (µg)	1.2

3 hours as frequent suckling stimulates the milk supply. Once lactation is well established, feeds can be spaced further apart.

Support for the mother from family, friends and health professionals is essential during the early weeks after delivery. The mother may become very tired, and practical help with housework and shopping is important.

Complementary feeding

This is the term used when infant formula milks are given in addition to breast feeding. This may be done for reasons of convenience or if the mother's milk supply is inadequate. However, complementary feeding diminishes the mother's milk supply even further, and a return to full breast feeding will be difficult. If complementary feeds are used at all, they should be offered after the breast feed.

Storage of breast milk

If the mother returns to work, there is no need for the infant to stop having breast milk. Mothers may partially breast feed the infant in the morning and the evening, say, and express milk for use by the infant's carer during the day.

Breast milk may be expressed manually or with a breast pump. Strict attention to hygiene is essential. Once the milk has been collected, it can be stored for up to 24 hours in a refrigerator and up to 3 months in a freezer.

Dietary supplements

In general the mother does not need to take dietary supplements, but if there is any doubt about the mother's diet, vitamin drops may be prescribed for the baby from the age of 1 month.

Problems with breast feeding

Mothers with difficulties in breast feeding may sometimes visit pharmacies with the intention of starting the infant on formula milk. Pharmacists should refer all such mothers to their health visitor or midwife before selling an infant milk.

Inadequate milk

The most common difficulty in breast feeding is the inadequate supply of milk and consequent failure of the infant to thrive. A number of factors may be responsible including illness and tiredness in the mother, and also tension or lack of confidence in feeding. The best way of increasing the milk supply is to increase the frequency of breast feeding, to encourage the mother to relax and take as much rest as possible, and to make sure that her diet is adequate.

Inverted nipples

About 10% of pregnant women intending to breast feed have inverted nipples, and this may lead to problems in establishing and maintaining breast feeding. Traditionally such women have been advised to prepare their breasts during pregnancy by the use of breast shells or Hoffman's exercises.

Breast shells consist of a saucer with a central orifice through which the nipple is inserted. A plastic cup fits over the saucer and a firm bra is worn over the top. Hoffman's exercises aim to stretch the nipples by manipulation.

There are conflicting views on the use of these techniques and there is no clear evidence that either method improves the chances of successful breast feeding. Neither technique should be recommended without medical referral.

Sore and cracked nipples

Sore nipples occur as a result of incorrectly positioning the baby at the breast. The baby should never be allowed to suck at the nipple itself but the nipple should be pushed right into the baby's mouth so that he or she is sucking not just on the nipple but also on the areola. If cracked nipples do occur, a nipple shield (not to be confused with a breast shield) may be worn and held in place while the infant feeds through it.

Breast engorgement, blocked ducts and mastitis

These conditions are painful and distressing for the mother, and all may be caused by incorrect positioning of the baby at the breast or by infrequent feeding. Mastitis may lead to breast abscesses, and early recognition and treatment are important. All mothers with these conditions should be referred to the doctor or health visitor.

Breast abscesses

This is a rare problem but it may occur if mastitis is left untreated. The mother should be referred to the doctor without delay. Breast abscesses may be treated with antibiotics but occasionally surgery may also be needed.

Bottle feeding

Despite encouragement to breast feed, some mothers choose to bottle feed and their decision should be respected. In addition some mothers may be unable to breast feed.

The advantages and disadvantages of bottle feeding

The advantages and disadvantages of bottle feeding are almost exactly the converse of those mentioned for breast feeding.

Advantages

(1) Other members of the family and friends can feed the baby; it is less tying for the mother and may create less jealousy in other family members.
(2) The volume of milk consumed can be seen.
(3) It creates no problems for the working mother.
(4) The milk supply is easily established.
(5) It creates no extra additional nutritional demands on the mother.

Disadvantages

(1) Although nutritionally adequate, it does not completely mimic the nutritional properties of breast milk.
(2) It gives no protection against infection.
(3) It contains potential allergens; infants may be allergic to cow's milk.
(4) It is more expensive than breast feeding.
(5) It requires careful preparation and storage.

(6) It may give less protection against chronic disease in later life.
(7) It provides no advantages to the mother in terms of weight reduction or uterus returning to normal.
(8) It may reduce mother–infant bonding.
(9) It has no contraceptive effect.

Types of infant feeds

Infant feeds are available in the form of powders for reconstitution, concentrates and ready-to-feed liquids. There are seven different types of infant feed and their nutrient composition is shown in Table 16.2. They are:

- Whey-based milks
- Casein-based milks
- Follow-on milks
- Pre-term milks
- Soya-based formulas
- Pre-digested milks
- Lactose-free, casein-based feeds

Whey-based milks

Whey-based milks most closely mimic breast milk, and mothers wishing to bottle feed should generally be advised to use them. There are no significant differences between the brands of these milks.

They are made by removing the fat, curd protein and mineral from cow's milk to produce demineralised whey. Skimmed or semi-skimmed milk, vegetable oils and vitamins are then added. They contain a whey:casein ratio of about 60:40 which is similar to that of breast milk.

Casein-based milks

The type of protein in cow's milk (i.e. casein) is not changed to make casein-based milks, but the quantity is reduced as is the concentration of sodium, potassium and chloride. This is achieved by the addition of vegetable fat and carbohydrate, in the form of lactose, maltodextrin and sucrose. The whey:-casein ratio is 20:80 and is similar to cow's milk. Like whey-based milks casein-based milks may be used from birth.

Many mothers change from one type of milk to another, and the use of casein-based milks increases steadily as the baby grows older. This is because many people believe that casein-based milks satisfy hunger better than a whey-based milk. Casein is relatively indigestible compared with whey, so it may provide an increased sense of satiety, but there is little evidence for this.

Follow-on milks

Follow-on milks differ from whey-and casein-based milks in that they

Table 16.2 Composition of infant milks (per 100 ml).

Milk or formula	Energy kJ(kcal)	CHO [g]	Fat [g]	Pr [g]	Prescribable indications
Whey-based infant milks[1]					
Aptamil (Milupal)	281 (67)	7.3	3.6	1.5	
First Milk (Farley)	284 (68)	7.0	3.8	1.5	
Formula 1 (Boots)	281 (77)	7.2	3.6	1.5	
Premium (Cow & Gate Nutricia)	277 (66)	7.5	3.5	1.4	
SMA Gold Cap (SMA Nutrition)	273 (65)	7.2	3.6	1.5	
Casein-based infant milks[1]					
Milumil (Milupa)	290 (69)	8.4	3.1	1.9	
Plus (Cow & Gate Nutricia)	280 (67)	7.3	3.4	1.7	
Second Milk (Farley)	277 (66)	8.3	2.9	1.7	
SMA White Cap (SMA Nutrition)	280 (67)	7.0	3.6	1.6	
Follow-on milks[1]					
Follow-on milk (Boots)	290 (69)	7.2	3.6	2.1	
Follow-on milk (Farley)	285 (68)	8.0	3.1	2.1	
Forward (Milupa)	295 (70)	7.2	3.6	2.0	
Progress (Wyeth)	281 (67)	7.8	3.0	2.2	
Stepup (Cow & Gate Nutricia)	295 (70)	8.0	3.4	1.8	
Pre-term infant milks[1]					
Prematil with Milupan (Milupa)	298 (70)	7.7	3.5	2.0	
Premcare (Farley)	301 (72)	7.2	4.0	1.9	
Prescribable feeds					
Soya-based formulas[1]					All for proven lactose interolerance in pre-school children, galactokinase deficiency, galactosaemia and proven whole cow's milk sensitivity
Farley's Soya Formula (Farley)	294 (70)	7.0	3.8	2.9	
Infasoy (Cow & Gate Nutricia)	280 (66)	7.1	3.6	1.8	
Isomil (Abbott)	286 (68)	6.9	3.7	1.8	
Prosobee (Bristol-Myers)	277 (65)	6.9	3.6	2.1	
Wysoy (SMA Nutrition)	281 (67)	6.9	3.6	2.1	

Cont.

Table 16.2 Cont.

Milk or formula	Energy kJ(kcal)	CHO [g]	Fat [g]	Pr [g]	Prescribable indications
Pre-digested feeds					
Alfare (Nestlé)	272 (65)	7.0	3.3	2.2	Disaccharide and whole protein intolerance, or where amino acids or peptides are indicated in conjunction with medium chain triglycerides (MCT)
MCT Pepdite 0–2 (Scientific Hospital Supplies)	277 (66)	8.9	2.7	2.1	Disorders in which a high intake of MCT is beneficial
Neocate (Scientific Hospital Supplies)	298 (71)	8.4	3.5	2.0	Proven whole protein intolerance, short bowel syndrome, intractable malabsorption, proven inflammatory bowel disease and bowel fistulas
Nutramigen (Bristol-Myers)	273 (65)	9.1	2.6	1.9	Disaccharide and/or whole protein intolerance where additional MCT is indicated
Pepdite 0–2 (Scientific Hospital Supplies)	277 (66)	8.9	2.7	2.1	Disaccharide and/or whole protein intolerance, or where amino acids or peptides are indicated in conjunction with MCT
Pepti-Junior (Cow & Gate)	280 (66)	7.2	3.7	2.0	Disaccharide and/or whole protein intolerance, or where amino acids or peptides are indicated in conjunction with MCT
Pregestimil (Bristol-Myers)	277 (66)	9.1	2.7	1.9	Disaccharide and/or whole protein intolerance or where amino acids or peptides are indicated in conjunction with MCT
Prejomin (Milupa)	315 (75)	8.6	3.6	2.0	Disaccharide and/or whole protein intolerance where additional MCT is indicated
Lactose-free, casein-based feeds					
AL110 (Nestlé)	280 (67)	7.4	3.3	1.9	Proven lactose intolerance in pre-school children, galactosaemia and galactokinase deficiency
Galactomin 17 (Scientific Hospital Supplies)	277 (66)	7.4	3.4	1.9	Proven lactose intolerance in pre-school children, galactosaemia and galactokinase deficiency
Galactomin 19 (Scientific Hospital Supplies)	228 (55)	7.3	1.8	2.8	Glucose plus galactose intolerance

[1] Suitable for vegetarians, but not those who avoid all animal products.
[2] Suitable for vegans.
CHO = Carbohydrate; Pr = protein.

contain a higher concentration of protein and electrolytes. They also contain more iron and vitamin D than either whey-and casein-based milks or cow's milk. They are designed for use in infants over 6 months old and should not be used for younger babies.

There is no need to change a baby's feed to this type of milk at 6 months old. Breast milk or whey-or casein-based milks can be continued until the baby is 12 months old.

However, iron deficiency is a risk in infants of 6 months and older because iron stored by the infant before birth will be depleted. Provided the infant is weaned on to a mixed diet containing iron-rich foods (see Appendix 3) the risk of deficiency is minimal. But, as everybody knows, toddlers can be incredibly faddy eaters, and if a nutritionally adequate diet is not achieved a follow-on milk may be of benefit. Follow-on milks may also be of benefit in Asian infants who are often found to be deficient in vitamin D.

Pre-term milks

Pre-term milks are intended to supply the extra nutritional needs of pre-mature babies. Most of these milks are only available in hospital but some are available in community pharmacies. Premature infants are usually fed on pre-term milks, either as a supplement to breast milk or as the sole source of nutrition, until the baby reaches about 2 kg in weight. The infant may then be breast or bottle fed.

Soya-based formulas

Soya-based formulas do not mimic breast milk as closely as either whey-or casein-based formulas. Some nutrients are less well absorbed from soya formulas, and they should only be used after referral to a doctor or dietitian. Casual use of these formulas as a replacement for regular infant milks should be discouraged.

Soya-based formulas are prescribable for lactose intolerance, proven whole cow's milk sensitivity, galactokinase deficiency and galactosaemia. For a description of these conditions see Chapter 9. Soya protein is not necessarily any less allergenic than cow's milk protein, and a pre-digested milk may be a better choice.

Pharmacists should not recommend these formulas to parents who believe their infant has an allergy unless the allergy has been properly diagnosed by a doctor in which case the formula will usually be prescribed. Nor should they be recommended for infants who have a family history of allergic conditions. Although soya formulas may be used for this purpose, medical advice should be sought first to establish the degree of potential risk.

Pre-digested milks and formulas

These products contain hydrolysed protein which needs minimal digestion, and they are lactose-free. The source of the protein may be either cow's milk or soya. They are prescribable for special purposes, such as disaccharide and whole protein intolerance. They are hypoallergenic and preferable to whole protein products – either cow's milk or soya – for the treatment of intolerances.

Like soya formulas pre-digested products should not be recommended by pharmacists without medical referral.

Lactose-free, casein-based feeds

These milks differ from the pre-digested formulas in that they contain casein which is unhydrolysed. They are prescribable for a range of disorders including lactose intolerance.

Preparation of feeds

Reconstitution

Correct preparation and reconstitution of infant feeds is essential and pharmacists should make sure that parents understand this (see box below). Over-concentrated feeds can cause dehydration and lead to obesity in the long term. Over-dilute feeds can lead to inadequate intake of nutrients and failure to thrive. Care should be taken not to swap scoops between different brands and not to pack the milk powder into the scoop. The powder should always be added to the bottle after the water has been added and not the other way round. A day's feeds can be made at one time, but they must be stored at the back of the refrigerator ready for use. The door compartments should not be used as the temperature may be too high, encouraging bacterial growth. Any unused milk should be thrown away after 24 hours.

General guidelines for preparation and use of infant feeds.

(1) Boil all feeding utensils (bottles, teats, rings, scoops) for 10 minutes before using
(2) Boil water in a separate vessel and pour the required quantity of hot (about 60°C) water into a feeding bottle
(3) Measure the correct number of scoops into the bottle and ensure that scoops are level
(4) Cap bottle and shake vigorously
(5) Check the temperature before feeding by shaking a few drops on the inside of the wrist. Allow to cool if too hot

---

Water

Feeds should be made up with domestic drinking water. The kettle should be freshly filled, boiled and then allowed to cool to about 60°C. Repeatedly boiled water should not be used as repeated evaporation may lead to over-concentration of minerals.

Water from a water-softened supply should not be used because the sodium content may be higher than from water drawn directly from the mains. Parents who use water filters should be warned to change these regularly, because of the potential risk of microbiological contamination.

Bottled waters should not be used routinely for reconstituting feeds, because many of them contain a high concentration of minerals. If parents are anxious about the purity of the tap water, e.g. when travelling abroad, then a bottled water of low sodium content, e.g. Evian, Highland Spring, Spa or Volvic, may be used. Like tap water, bottled water should always be boiled before use in the preparation of infant feeds.

Microwaves

Microwave ovens should not be used to warm up infant feeds. Although the bottle of milk may feel the right temperature, there is a risk of scalding the baby because the temperature at the centre of the milk is too high. Moreover, microwaving does not sterilise bottles, teats or other feeding equipment. These should be sterilised by the use of chemicals or by boiling.

Problems associated with feeding

Common problems related to feeding include wind, vomiting, colic, constipation, diarrhoea and various intolerances.

Wind

Wind is more likely to be a problem in infants who are bottle fed than those who are breast fed. This is because they tend to take in more air. Wind can be minimised by stopping the baby from feeding at intervals and allowing him or her to rest in a vertical position so that the air can escape.

Vomiting

Regurgitation of small amounts of feed is common in both breast and bottle fed infants. If a large proportion of the milk is repeatedly being regurgitated, the infant should be referred to the doctor.

Colic

Colic should not be confused with wind. Symptoms are more severe and include abdominal pain and crying or screaming. It usually starts during the first month of the infant's life and may continue until the age of 3 months. It occurs in both breast and bottle fed infants.

Infants with suspected colic should be referred to the doctor. Once a diagnosis has been made, reassurance that the baby is normal and that the condition will gradually resolve may be all that is necessary. Anti-spasmodic drugs may help some infants.

Colic in breast fed infants may be caused by dairy products in the mother's diet and the mother may be advised to try avoiding these foods. For bottle fed infants a lactose-free formula may be tried. If these changes are effective, substantial improvement will occur within a week.

Constipation

Stools may be passed irregularly in both breast and bottle fed babies, but so long as the stool is soft the infant is not constipated. Constipation is more likely to occur in a bottle fed infant, and may be caused by an inadequate fluid intake. Cooled, boiled water should be offered to bottle fed infants between feeds particularly in hot weather.

Once the infant is over 3 months of age, fruit juice should be given but bran products should be avoided.

Diarrhoea

Diarrhoea is most commonly caused by viral infection. Infants under 3 months old should always be referred to the doctor, and infants of any age with prolonged diarrhoea of more than 24 hours' duration should also be referred.

Oral rehydration therapy

Replacement of lost fluids is the single most important factor in treating diarrhoea in both infants and adults. A variety of oral rehydration solutions exist for this purpose and sachets rather than tablets should be recommended for infants under 1 year old.

Pharmacists should make sure that parents understand the importance of following manufacturers' instructions, since incorrectly prepared solutions may result in electrolyte imbalance. Freshly boiled and cooled water should always be used for the preparation of oral rehydration solutions in infants. A volume which is one to one and a half times the usual feed volume is recommended for children under 2 years of age, but an infant who wants more to drink can be given extra solution.

Home-made sugar and salt solutions should not be used, and water should not be given without electrolytes because of the danger of water intoxication.

Feeding

In both breast and bottle fed infants, feeding should continue in addition to oral rehydration therapy. The widespread practice of diluting bottle feeds should be discouraged. Dilution has no beneficial effect on the course of the illness and, contrary to previous thinking, it does not reduce the risk of lactose intolerance. Reducing milk intake when it is the infant's only source of food may cause weight loss.

Infants who have been weaned may continue taking solid food if they have the appetite. Small meals of bland foods are the best choice.

Drugs

Drugs, including antibiotics and antidiarrhoeals, have no role in the management of diarrhoea of viral origin.

Intolerance conditions

Infants may be intolerant to feeds because of disaccharide intolerance, cow's milk protein sensitivity or various inborn errors of metabolism (see Chapter 9).

Weaning

Weaning means introducing a baby to foods other than milk. It is a gradual process which can take weeks or months.

Weaning is necessary because nutritional requirements can no longer be met by milk alone. The volume of milk produced is unlikely to meet energy requirements, and iron stores which were built up by the infant before birth become depleted. Once teeth are present, feeding behaviour progresses from sucking to biting and chewing.

Age

The age at which babies are ready to take solid food varies, and a flexible approach should be adopted, but weaning should generally not start before 3 months of age nor should it be delayed beyond 6 months.

Solids should not be introduced too early, because the infant is unable to bite and chew and the gastrointestinal tract is more vulnerable to infections and possibly to intolerance conditions such as coeliac disease. On the other hand, late weaning may result in depleted iron stores and anaemia.

Starting weaning

Solids should be given by spoon and never added to bottles. New foods should be offered one at a time, and 1–2 teaspoons is enough at first. At this stage getting the baby used to the idea of eating solid food is more important than its nutrient content, but the aim of weaning is to encourage the infant to eat a healthy diet, and a wide range of nutritious foods should be offered as soon as possible.

Suitable weaning foods are shown in Table 16.3.

Table 16.3 Weaning foods.

Age	Suitable foods	Foods to avoid
3–6 months	Baby rice; vegetable purées (carrots, yams, potatoes, plantain, cauliflower, swede, green vegetables); fruit purées (apple, pear, banana); puréed lentils; porridge (made from cornmeal, sago or millet) Gradually include puréed lean meat (including liver), poultry and fish	Eggs, wheat foods, citrus fruits, nuts, sugar, salt
6–9 months	Yoghurt, cottage cheese, bread, toast, chapattis, naans, egg yolks, citrus fruits, smooth peanut butter	Sugar, salt, whole nuts
10–12 months	Introduce family meals	

Food preparation

Initially all foods offered to the infant must be mashed or sieved. A food processor may be used for this purpose. At about 6 months foods with a rougher texture containing small lumps may be offered. Babies of 8–10 months should be offered chunks of food, for example small pieces of unpeeled carrot or apple.

Sterilisation of feeds and equipment is not essential once weaning has started but attention to hygiene in the preparation of food for infants is important.

Sugar and salt should not be added to infants' foods. Regular use of salt may lead to hypernatraemia, and sugar encourages a sweet tooth which may cause dental caries and obesity.

Commercial foods

Commercial foods are available in the form of powders for reconstitution and ready-to-feed jars and tins. They can be classified into three broad groups:

- Baby rice products
- Foods to be used from the age of 3–4 months (sometimes called Stage 1 foods)
- Foods to be used from the age of 6–7 months (sometimes called Stage 2 or Junior foods)

Within these groups there are a variety of types of main meal, dessert, yoghurt and fruit. Commercial foods are available in gluten-free, sugar-free, milk-free, egg-free and vegetarian varieties. Many are also free of additives, colours and preservatives.

Commercial foods have a useful role in weaning, particularly of infants whose families have poor diets. They are not nutritionally inferior to home-prepared foods. Dried foods are particularly useful at first, because small amounts can be made up and the rest of the packet kept. Once opened, foods from jars and cans must be kept in the fridge and foods should never be left in opened cans.

The main drawback of commercial foods is that they delay or discourage the introduction of family meals. They are also expensive.

Milk

Breast milk, or a suitable infant milk or formula, should be continued until the infant is 12 months old, but it should not be used as the sole source of nutrition after 6 months of age. The use of other milks will now be considered (see Table 16.4).

Table 16.4   Use of milks in infants and young children.

Age	Type of milk
Under 6 months	Breast or infant formula milk
6–12 months	Breast or infant formula milk; follow-on milk
Over 12 months	Whole cow's milk; semi-skimmed milk not recommended for children under 2 years; skimmed milk not recommended for children under 5 years

Cow's milk

Cow's milk is higher in protein and electrolytes and lower in iron than either breast milk or infant feeds. It is unsuitable for infants under 6 months of age and should preferably not be given to infants under 1 year of age. This is because cow's milk contains less iron than breast and infant milks.

Cow's milk is, however, an important part of a child's diet after 1 year and the consumption of one pint a day should be encouraged at least until the age of 5 years. Skimmed and semi-skimmed milks are not recommended for children under 5 years of age, but semi-skimmed milk may be introduced from 2 years of age provided the overall diet is adequate.

Soya milk

Unmodified soya milks sold for general use in health food shops and supermarkets should not be given to children under 5 years of age. They contain only soya beans and water, and sometimes sugar, and are nutritionally inadequate compared with cow's milk.

Modified soya infant formulas are suitable but should only be used under medical supervision.

Goat's and sheep's milk

Goat's and sheep's milk are sometimes used by parents in an attempt to prevent or treat cow's milk allergy. They are deficient in vitamins, particularly folic acid, and should not be used in children under 5 years of age.

Infant drinks

Infants who are thirsty should be encouraged to drink boiled, cooled water. Fruit juices and fruit drinks should not be given until the infant is 3 months old.

There is an increasing variety of infant drinks in the form of ready-to-feed liquids, concentrates and powders for reconstitution. Many are labelled as being with 'no added sugar', but, as with foods and drinks for adults, this does not necessarily mean that the product contains no sugar. Most infant drinks contain glucose, dextrose or fructose. If fruit drinks are given to infants, care should always be taken to brush the teeth afterwards.

Unsweetened fruit juice may be given, but until the infant is 6 months old this should be diluted about one part in eight with water. Thereafter, until the infant is 12 months old, fruit juice should be diluted about one in four.

Healthy eating after weaning

The principles of healthy eating for adults are not appropriate for infants. This is because infants have greater energy and nutrient requirements for their size than adults. Too much emphasis on foods low in fat and high in non-starch polysaccharides (NSP) may prejudice energy intake. NSP-rich foods tend to be bulky which may mean that the infant's appetite is satisfied from a lower energy intake than is required for growth. Although wholemeal bread should be offered to infants and young children, bran should be avoided.

Iron deficiency is one of the main nutritional problems of infants and toddlers, and iron-rich foods should be emphasised in the diet from about 4–6 months (see Appendix 3). Some brands of infant rusks (e.g. Farleys) are also rich in iron.

Dietary supplements

Multivitamins

Apart from vitamin K, infants under the age of 6 months do not generally need dietary supplements. Both breast and infant milks normally provide sufficient vitamins and minerals. However, if the mother of a breast fed infant has a poor diet, the infant may be at risk of deficiency, and vitamin drops may be recommended from the age of 1 month.

The need for extra vitamins is more likely to arise when the infant is weaned. The Department of Health recommends that all infants and young children be given children's vitamin drops from the age of 6 months until 5 years unless the infant is considered to be obtaining enough vitamin A from the diet and enough vitamin D from the diet and/or sunlight. Generic vitamin drops are available direct to the public from maternity and child health clinics. Proprietary brands (e.g. Abidec and Adexolin) are available from pharmacies.

Vitamin K

Vitamin K deficiency may occur soon after birth because the gut is sterile and normal vitamin K synthesis does not occur. Vitamin K is given to prevent haemorrhagic disease in newborn infants. Parenteral administration of vitamin K has been associated in some studies with an increased risk of cancer in childhood but later studies have not confirmed these findings. A joint MCA (Medicines Control Agency), CSM (Committee on Safety of Medicines) and DoH (Department of Health) expert group has concluded that overall, the available data do not support an increased risk of cancer, including leukaemia, caused by vitamin K.

Further reading

Davies, D.P. (1995) *Nutrition in Child Health*. Royal College of Physicians, London.

Department of Health (1994) Weaning and the weaning diet. Report on Health and Social Subjects No 45. HMSO, London.

MAFF (1997) *Healthy Diets for Infants and Young Children*. Ministry of Agriculture, Fisheries and Food, London.

Thomas, M. & Avery, V. (1997) *Infant Feeding in Asian Families*. The Stationery Office, London.

Wharton, B. (1997) *Nutrition in Infancy*. British Nutrition Foundation, London.

Wharton, B. (1997) Weaning in Britain: Practice, Policy and Problems. *Proceedings of the Nutrition Society*, 56, 105–119.

Useful addresses

National Information for Parents of Prematures, Education, Research and Support (NIPPERS), PO Box 1553, Wedmore, Somerset, BS28 4LZ. Tel: 01934 713630.

Chapter 17
Children and Young People

Nutritional requirements from infancy to adulthood will be discussed in two parts: children, and young people (adolescents or teenagers).

Children

It is important to establish good dietary habits in childhood to lay the foundations for life-long healthy eating. This is not always easy, but every effort should be made. Clearly, dietary advice for children will need to be aimed at the parents or carers.

Pharmacists frequently dispense prescriptions for children, and parents often ask for advice about minor ailments. The incidence of infections and other conditions may be increased by poor diet, and pharmacists can do a great deal to encourage healthy eating in children.

Pre-school children

Young children are completely dependent on parents and carers for their meals, and will often want to imitate what is being eaten by the rest of the household. The presence of a young child can therefore be a time for the whole family to review their eating habits. Healthy eating habits will benefit the parents and help to set a good example to the young child.

As every parent knows, young children can be fussy eaters and with the best will in the world good eating patterns can be difficult to achieve. All too often mealtimes can be a battle ground, and, although this is distressing for parents, food should not be allowed to become an issue. No toddler can be forced to eat, and if a meal is refused it should be removed and food offered again at the next meal or snack time. On no account should sweets be offered instead. Children may eat erratically for days or weeks but they seldom go hungry.

School children

Once children start school, they tend to become more independent and have more autonomy over their food intake. Since 1980 there has been no requirement for schools to provide midday meals except for children from low-income families, and many children now have packed lunches. Some schools operate cash cafeterias and tuck shops, which all too often provide food that is low in essential nutrients and too high in fat and sugar.

Parents should be encouraged to find out what their children are eating while at school and to plan the other meals accordingly.

Nutritional requirements

Like adults, children need energy and nutrients to repair and maintain body tissues, and also for activity. Growth imposes extra demands, metabolic rate is high and young children are usually extremely active. Not surprisingly, children have much higher energy and nutrient requirements for their size than adults.

The Dietary Reference Values for children of different ages can be found in Appendix 1. It should be remembered that these are average values for groups of children and not individual needs. Individual requirements will vary considerably.

Healthy eating

Healthy eating in childhood is important not only because it affects the growth and development of the child but also because some disease processes, for example dental caries, obesity and cardiovascular disease, may start quite early in life.

Dietary guidelines for adults are not entirely appropriate for young children. Whereas a diet which is high in non-starch polysaccharides (NSP) and low in fat is a healthy choice for an inactive overweight adult, it may not provide sufficient energy for an active growing child.

On the type of diet recommended for healthy adults young children would have to eat twice their normal volume of food in order to satisfy their energy requirements. But young children have small stomachs and are unable to consume such large amounts of food in one sitting, so should instead be offered frequent small meals and snacks.

Breakfast is an important meal for young children. During recent years eating has become more informal and breakfast is a meal that many people may skip. There is of course no need for breakfast or for any 'proper' meal in the traditional sense, but breakfast provides energy and nutrients that, if missed, must be made up later in the day. Prolonging the time without food makes it more likely that a child – or an adult for that matter – will snack on sugary foods in the middle of the morning. The breakfast does not need to be a cooked one: cereals, milk, fruit juice and toast are quite adequate.

Children tend to eat from a more limited range of foods than adults. Since they have relatively high nutrient needs, the diet should be based on as many nutrient-dense foods as possible, e.g. milk, meat, poultry, fish, cheese, eggs, yoghurt, pulses, bread, cereals, fruit and vegetables. Most children enjoy sweets but these should not be eaten every day.

Fat

Fat is important in the diet of young children, and emphasis should not be given to too many low fat foods. This does not mean that children should eat large quantities of fried foods, but low fat spreads are not necessary.

Skimmed milk should not be given to children under 5 years, but semi-skimmed milk can be used from the age of 2 years provided the rest of the diet is adequate.

Non-starch polysaccharides (NSP)

There are no Dietary Reference Values for NSP in young children. The point has already been made that young children find it difficult to obtain enough energy from a diet which is bulky and high in NSP. Nevertheless, NSP is important in the diet of a young child, and constipation may occur if the diet contains very little. The best advice is to offer bulky foods such as fruit after meals or as between-meal snacks, when energy requirements have been satisfied.

From the age of about 5–7 years NSP intake should gradually be increased by encouraging the child to eat more wholemeal bread, wholegrain cereals and fruit and vegetables.

Sugar

The consumption of sugar is related to dental caries and should be restricted.

Dietary advice in childhood.

(1) Food intake should maintain activity and height and weight in the desirable range

(2) Overweight and obesity should be corrected by reducing weight gain and allowing height to catch up with weight rather than by aiming for weight loss

(3) Overemphasis on a diet high in NSP and low in fat should be avoided; such a diet may be too bulky to provide a child's energy requirements

(4) Children under 5 years should normally drink 1 pint of whole cow's milk a day. Skimmed milk should be avoided under 5 years of age. Semi-skimmed milk may be introduced after 2 years

(5) Frequent small meals and snacks, including breakfast, should be encouraged

(6) Emphasis should be given to a diet rich in nutrient-dense foods such as meat, poultry, fish, milk, cheese, eggs, bread, cereals, fruit and vegetables

(7) Sweets should be restricted to once or twice a week or on special occasions; they should not be used as rewards

(8) Children's vitamin drops should be taken from 6 months until 5 years

Nutritional problems

The major nutritional problems associated with childhood are dental decay, iron deficiency, vitamin D deficiency, weight control, food allergy and hyperactivity.

Dental caries

Dental caries are common in children although the incidence has fallen considerably during recent years. This is mainly due to better oral hygiene and fluoridation of water supplies. The intake of sugary foods has not changed.

Children are particularly susceptible to dental caries when their permanent teeth are erupting. Of course it is impossible to prevent children from eating sweets entirely, and the best approach is to limit their intake to once or twice a week or on special occasions. Sweets should not be eaten every day and should not be offered as rewards.

Some sweets cause more damage than others, particularly toffees which tend to stick to the teeth and boiled sweets which are sucked for prolonged periods. Chocolate is less cariogenic. Children should always be encouraged to brush their teeth after eating sweets.

If the level of fluoride in the drinking water is low, fluoride supplements may be recommended (see Chapter 8).

Iron deficiency

Iron deficiency is fairly common in young children. It is a particular risk in those from low income families and those of Asian origin. Iron is best absorbed from animal food sources such as red meat, but less so from plant sources. Vitamin C promotes the absorption of iron from plant foods such as wheat and cereals, and a glass of fruit juice is a useful addition to each meal, particularly for vegetarians.

Green vegetables are good sources of both iron and vitamin C and should be encouraged – that is, if the child will eat them. Many children claim to loathe green vegetables!

Vitamin D deficiency

Deficiency of vitamin D causes rickets in children (see Chapter 13).

Weight control

Weight and height gain in young children normally fluctuate, but so long as height and weight compare favourably with standard reference curves all is likely to be well.

Obesity and overweight are becoming significant problems in an increasing number of children. By the age of 11 years about 18% of the population are overweight. The risk of obese children becoming obese adults has been extensively debated, but unless obesity is severe in childhood there appears to be a poor correlation between childhood and adult obesity. What is more likely is that children with obese parents will become overweight themselves. This may be a genetic problem, or it may be due to the inheritance of unhealthy eating patterns.

If weight does need to be reduced, dietary changes should be gentle and gradual. Drastic energy reduction can induce changes in eating behaviour that do more harm than good. In children the aim should be to reduce weight gain and to allow height to catch up with weight, rather than to encourage actual weight loss.

Food intolerance

Food intolerance is described in Chapter 9.

Hyperactivity

Many parents believe that their child is hyperactive, but bad behaviour in children is multifactorial and need not necessarily be blamed on food. Some food additives are associated with hyperactivity (see Chapter 4). Diagnosis by parents is not always reliable and a doctor's opinion should be sought. If hyperactivity due to food is diagnosed, the offending item or items should be removed from the diet under the supervision of a dietitian.

The idea that chemicals added to food cause hyperactivity is the basis of the Feingold diet. This diet eliminates all food and drink containing artificial colour and flavouring and also all fruits and vegetables containing natural salicylates. Other items excluded are toothpaste, aspirin, and most other medications including vitamins. In addition to Feingold's original diet other additives, such as monosodium glutamate, nitrates, butylated hydroxytoluene and butylated hydroxyanisole, may be excluded. Despite the lack of evidence that such diets work, they remain quite popular.

Dietary supplements

The majority of children do not need extra vitamins, but it is recognised that some children's diets are poor and they are at risk of deficiency. The Department of Health recommends children's vitamin drops for all children until 5 years of age, unless the diet is known to be adequate. Children's vitamin drops are available from child clinics, and equivalent proprietary brands (e.g. Abidec and Adexolin) from pharmacies.

Intelligence

There has been a great deal of debate about the influence of dietary supplements on childhood intelligence. Adequate nutrient intake is important for mental performance, and supplements may improve mental performance in malnourished children. However, vitamin supplements are not a panacea for increasing intelligence in schoolchildren.

Young people

This section describes the nutritional needs of young people (adolescents) between childhood and adulthood, and broadly covers the teenage years. Pharmacists do not have a great deal of contact with this age group through dispensing, and perhaps the most obvious opportunity to give dietary advice to young people is when they ask for advice about acne and skin products. In contrast to what many people believe, acne is not caused by fatty foods.

Adolescence is a time of great physiological and psychological change. Physiological changes influence nutritional requirements, and psychological changes tend to affect eating patterns.

Physiological changes include a marked acceleration in growth and gain in bone and muscle tissue. During the growth spurt, boys gain on average about 20 cm in height and girls about 10 cm. Boys gain proportionately more muscle and bone and girls more fat.

For most boys and girls the teenage years are a period of increasing independence from the family, and often a time of rebellion. Nowadays many young people have a great deal of control over what they eat, but busy schedules at school or college and the influence of friends may mean that food choices are not always the healthiest.

Advertisements directed at young people as well as children tend to be for foods high in fat and sugar. A quick glance at a teenage magazine or a few television advertisements during children's prime viewing time will confirm this. But what impact such advertising has on eating habits is difficult to assess.

Nutritional concerns in young people tend to be related to weight loss and body shape, complexion and environmental issues. Adolescence is a time of growing social awareness, and vegetarianism is becoming increasingly popular in this age group.

Nutritional requirements

The demand for energy and nutrients increases during adolescence. Nutritional requirements for young people of different ages are shown in Appendix 1.

Energy

Energy requirements are highest during the growth spurt, but the need for energy should not be overestimated. The estimated average requirement (EAR) for energy in 15- to 18-year-old boys is only 1.1 MJ (200 kcal) higher than for an adult male. The corresponding figure for girls is 0.7 MJ (170 kcal). Many young people seem to be permanently hungry and should be encouraged to 'fill up' with foods rich in complex carbohydrates, such as bread and cereals. Energy requirements also depend on physical activity; some teenagers are relatively inactive whilst others take part in regular sport.

Protein

The range of protein requirements for teenagers varies between 42 and 55 g a day. These quantities can easily be met by the average diet so there is no need to emphasise protein intake in the diet of young people.

Iron

The need for iron increases in boys as well as girls. it is required in both sexes for the increase in lean body mass, blood volume and haemoglobin as well as for menstrual losses in girls.

Calcium

Calcium is particularly important in young people. The risk of developing osteoporosis is related to the level of peak bone mass achieved and whilst this is not reached until the middle of the third decade, approximately 45% of the skeleton is laid down during adolescence.

Positive calcium balance and a healthy skeleton are promoted by weight-bearing physical exercise, and young people should be encouraged to increase activities such as walking, dancing, running and racquet sports.

Eating habits

There is a trend in society away from conventional foods and meal patterns towards more informal eating habits, including take-aways and snacks. Teenagers and young adults currently reflect these trends probably more than any other age group. Such eating habits are not necessarily harmful. Adequate nutrient intake is not dependent on 'proper' meals, but the diets of many teenagers do tend to be high in fatty and sugary foods and low in fruit and vegtetables.

Nutritional problems

Many young people's diets tend to be high in fat and sugar and low in NSP. Iron intake may be low, particularly in girls, and calcium intake may be low in both sexes. Other nutritional problems are related to weight control, pregnancy and fundamental changes in eating habits such as vegetarianism. Smoking and excessive alcohol intake will also prejudice nutrient status.

Iron deficiency

Adolescent girls who have started to menstruate are at greater risk of iron deficiency than boys. Iron-rich foods should be emphasised (see Appendix 3), and an iron supplement should be recommended if the girl's periods are heavy.

Calcium deficiency

Young people's diets may be deficient in calcium, and the importance of calcium-rich foods (see Appendix 4) cannot be overemphasised in this age group. A pint of milk a day goes some way towards meeting calcium requirements, and this may be skimmed or semi-skimmed particularly for teenagers who are concerned about their weight.

Calcium supplements may be recommended for teenagers who refuse to eat calcium-rich foods.

Weight control

The teenage years are often a time of concern about weight and shape. While boys may worry about gaining enough muscle mass, girls are often concerned about gaining too much fat. At the age of 14 about 18% of males and 22% of females are either obese or overweight, but about one-third of boys and two-thirds of girls at this age have tried 'dieting' to lose or avoid gaining weight.

In young people who are slimming there is a risk of multiple deficiencies including calcium, iron, vitamin A, vitamin B_6, folate and riboflavin as well as a risk of developing anorexia nervosa or bulimia nervosa. For young people who really do need to watch their weight, it is better to recommend an increase in physical activity and a moderate reduction in energy intake.

Pregnancy

The combined stresses of pregnancy and adolescence may prove to be a great physical and psychological burden. The risks of nutrient deficiency in adolescence are increased because it is likely that stores of nutrients will be low.

Demands for calcium, iron, zinc and folate will be particularly high, and the importance of obtaining energy from nutrient-dense foods should be stressed.

Vegetarianism

Increasing awareness about social and environmental issues may lead young people to vegetarianism. A well chosen vegetarian diet can be extremely healthy, but this is not always the case.

Young people at greatest risk of nutritional deficiency are likely to be those who eat family meals and avoid the meat dish without eating a substitute. This may be because of parental resistance to vegetarianism, and family acceptance will do much to help young people maintain a balanced vegetarian diet. Although this may involve some inconvenience in meal preparation, young people can be encouraged to prepare their own meat alternative and occasionally the whole family can eat a vegetarian meal. This may be of benefit to the whole family in terms of reducing fat intake.

Smoking and alcohol

Smoking and drinking habits in young people are a matter of concern. The prevalence of both activities increases with age, and by the age of 15 as many as a third of young people may be regular smokers. At the same age the majority are drinking some alcohol, but this is only worrying if the intake is particularly high, e.g. more than 7 units a week (see Chapter 3 for an explanation of alcohol units).

Smoking alters the metabolism of vitamin C, and excessive alcohol intake alters the absorption of many nutrients including thiamin, folic acid and vitamin C. Risks of deficiency will be even greater in those who are slimming.

Dietary advice

Young people may not be very receptive to dietary advice, not least because of their growing independence. Another factor is that at this age most individuals do not tend to think very far ahead, and talking about the risks of coronary heart disease in later life is likely to fall on deaf ears. With the right approach pharmacists and other health professionals may have more influence than parents and teachers.

Dietary advice for teenagers is basically the same as that for healthy adults, i.e. the diet should contain a variety of nutrient-dense foods, be rich in complex carbohydrates and NSP, and low in fat, sugar and salt. Account must be taken of the foods which teenagers are likely to eat, and the following suggestions to teenagers or their parents may be helpful:

- Jacket potatoes with low fat fillings such as baked beans or cottage cheese are healthier take-aways than chips or fries.
- Chips should be thick-cut and preferably oven-style, and low in fat or fried in polyunsaturated oil.
- Sandwiches and toast should be wholemeal.
- Fizzy drinks and squashes should be of the 'diet' or low sugar variety.
- Unsalted nuts, plain popcorn, bread sticks, pittas and currant buns are healthier snacks than sweets, chocolates and crisps.
- Milk can be used in milk shakes or hot chocolate: both can be made with skimmed or semi-skimmed milk.
- Burgers should be low fat or made with lean meat and grilled.
- Fruit and fruit juice consumption should be encouraged as much as possible.
- Vegetable dishes such as corn on the cob, coleslaw made with low calorie mayonnaise, and bean salads may be more acceptable than traditional vegetables.

Dietary supplements

Nutrient requirements can easily be met from a varied diet, and dietary supplements should not be necessary. Teenagers who cannot be persuaded to eat calcium-rich foods should take a calcium supplement, and girls who have heavy periods should take an iron supplement. Those who are slimming or vegetarians should take a multi-vitamin and mineral supplement.

Further reading

National Dairy Council (1995) Nutrition and Children Aged One to Five. Fact File No 2 (revised edition). The National Dairy Council, London.

National Dairy Council (1995) Nutrition and Teenagers. Fact File No 5 (revised edition). The National Dairy Council, London.

Sharp, I. (1992) Nutritional Guidelines for School Meals. Report of an Expert Working Group. The Caroline Walker Trust, London.

Useful addresses

Hyperactive Children's Support Group, 71 Whyke Lane, Chichester, West Sussex PO19 2LD. Tel: 01903 725182.

Chapter 18
The Elderly

The elderly are usually defined as those of pensionable age. There are currently about 10 million elderly people in the UK and the numbers, particularly of those aged over 80, are likely to increase.

This chapter focuses on nutritional problems faced by the elderly. It should be remembered that many old people eat well and are fit and active, but in general elderly people use the health and community services more than younger people, and pharmacists will be well aware of the number of prescriptions they dispense for patients in this age group. Some elderly people may be at risk of nutritional deficiencies.

Pharmacists can make a useful contribution to nutritional problems in the elderly, for example by watching for drug–nutrient interactions, and by keeping an eye out for early signs of malnutrition (see Chapter 27).

Nutritional requirements

Energy requirements tend to fall with age for two reasons. First, elderly people tend to be less active, and secondly the metabolic rate falls because of a decrease in the amount of muscle and lean tissue. These two factors are of course interlinked; if activity is reduced, so is the amount of muscle tissue.

Many elderly people do remain active and some may even be more active after retirement than before, because they were employed in a sedentary job. Thus, there may be little difference in the energy requirements of a 50- and a 70-year-old.

Although the requirement for energy m ay fall, the need for nutrients does not, and Dietary Reference Values for vitamins and minerals in the elderly (see Appendix 1) are no different from those in young and middle-aged adults. The only exception is iron in women; the need for iron falls after menstruation ceases.

The fact that energy requirements tend to fall and nutrient needs remain the same means that the quality of the diet is very important. In other words, dietary advice to elderly people needs to emphasise the importance of nutrient-dense foods.

Causes of poor nutrition

Poor nutrition in the elderly is more likely to be related to lack of interest in food and to not eating enough rather than to over-nutrition and obesity.

The causes of poor nutrition in old people can be divided into socio-economic, psychological and physical factors which are often interlinked. An awareness of these factors should alert pharmacists to the possibility of poor nutrition in their elderly customers. Malnutrition can be corrected more easily if detected early.

Socio-economic factors

Most people take a drop in income when they retire, and poverty, which is a greater risk in the lower social classes, can be a real problem. When there is a lack of money, food is often the first economy made. Lack of transport very often means that elderly people have to rely on corner shops, which tend to be more expensive than supermarkets. Small pack sizes tend to be less readily available than family packs, and are also far more expensive.

Psychological factors

The incidence of depression increases in elderly people. Feelings of useless-ness, isolation, or recent bereavement may cause elderly people to become depressed and apathetic. This may affect their motivation to cook and prepare food.

Physical factors

Although many elderly people are fit and well, the incidence of disease increases with age. Cardiovascular disease, diabetes mellitus and respiratory and musculoskeletal disorders are more common in the elderly. Patients with arthritis or Parkinson's disease or those who have had strokes are likely to have difficulties in preparing and eating food.

Missing teeth, badly fitting dentures and sore gums may make chewing uncomfortable. Many old people experience changes in taste, and this may reduce the appetite and prevent enjoyment of food.

Multiple drug regimens are commonly prescribed for the elderly, and drugs can interact with nutrition in several ways (see Chapter 26). Some may reduce appetite and lead to changes in taste as well as increase the risk of nutrient deficiency.

Nutritional advice

Elderly people should be encouraged to eat a healthy diet (see Chapter 3), but it is important that dietary advice is not given in such a way that they are put off their food. Losing interest in food is likely to do far more damage to health and well-being than eating cakes and biscuits.

Worrying about changing to a low fat spread after a lifetime of eating butter may do more harm than good. In any case, atherosclerosis is usually well advanced by this stage in life, and, although there is some evidence that it can be stopped or reversed, attempts to reduce the fat content of the diet may prejudice the intake of other nutrients and energy. Elderly people who are overweight may be better staying that way than becoming over-anxious about their diet, unless gross obesity is contributing to other health problems.

What some elderly people may need is help and advice which can make shopping, food preparation and eating easier. Elderly people do not always buy and prepare their own food. Relatives, neighbours and home helps may take responsibility for this, and it is they who will need help and advice. Meals-on-wheels deliver ready-made meals, and, by providing an opportunity to socialise, luncheon clubs may help to reduce a sense of isolation.

The social services may be able to help with adaptation of home equipment for food preparation and consumption. Heavy cutlery is useful for people with tremor, and light cutlery for those with poor lifting ability and grip strength. For those who eat slowly, a heated trolley can be helpful.

Store cupboards

The importance of a store of food should be stressed to elderly people, particularly if they are unable to shop regularly. Useful items for the store cupboard include:

- Packets of UHT and dried milk
- Cans and packets of soup
- Tinned meat and fish
- Sandwich pastes and spreads
- Cereals
- Fruit juice, tinned fruit and dried fruit
- Rice and pasta
- Biscuits and crackers
- Tea, coffee and drinking chocolate

The milkman can be a useful source of heavy grocery items such as bread, potatoes, fruit juice, yoghurt and eggs. For elderly people with arthritis in their hands, packets will be more useful than tins.

Meal replacements

Meal replacements such as Build-Up and Complan are useful adjuncts to the diet, particularly when a person cannot face ordinary food. They are nutritionally adequate, but they should not be used as the sole source of nutrition for prolonged periods (more than about 2 weeks) without medical supervision. One problem with meal replacements is boredom, so alternative flavours should be offered.

Dietary supplements

There should be no need for dietary supplements provided the diet is varied and enough food is consumed. However, many elderly people are unable to eat a healthy and varied diet, so recommending a multivitamin and mineral supplement is a wise precaution. Vitamin D supplements are important for those who are housebound.

Problems associated with nutrition

Nutrient deficiency

Some elderly people are at risk of vitamin deficiency because of a poor diet. Intake of vitamin C is frequently poor, so elderly people should be encouraged to eat plenty of fruit and vegetables.

If people become less mobile or housebound, it becomes increasingly difficult to obtain adequate vitamin D from the action of sunlight on the skin, especially in Northern Britain. Elderly people should be encouraged to expose some skin to sunlight regularly during the summer months. If this is not possible, vitamin D supplementation should be considered, especially during the winter and early spring. *helps Ca²⁺ absorption !*

recommended is 10 µg/day for women over 65 y old

Many elderly people are at risk of Vitamin B_{12} deficiency. This is due, in part, to reduced gastric acid secretion, and lack of intrinsic factor, which is vital for absorption of the vitamin.

Iron deficiency is common in this age group. It can be caused by poor dietary intake and by blood loss from gastrointestinal disorders or the use of certain drugs. Haem iron (e.g. from red meat) should be emphasised because it is well absorbed. However, for those who consume red meat infrequently or not at all, a source of vitamin C should be consumed with each meal of snack.

Calcium is also important in this age group, because it helps to maintain bone mass. Although calcium cannot restore tissue that has already been lost from the bone, it can slow bone loss. *recommended, 1500 mg/day) – elderly > 70y old, or susceptible to osteoporosis.*

Constipation

Constipation is a common problem in the elderly, often because of lack of food or exercise or both. It is essential to find out whether the problem is of long duration or of sudden onset and to consider the possibility of underlying disease. It is also important to establish what the person considers to be normal bowel habit.

The best advice is to increase the intake of non-starch polysaccharides (NSP) by eating more wholemeal bread, wholegrain cereals and fruit and *present consideration*

vegetables. Raw bran should be avoided because of its phytate content which may prejudice mineral absorption. Fluid intake should also be increased to about 8 cups a day and regular exercise such as walking should be encouraged if possible.

Osteoporosis

pg 123

Osteoporosis is described in Chapter 13. Emphasis should be given to calcium intake and exercise. it is particularly important to resume exercise promptly after periods of ill health.

Further reading

Caroline Walker Trust (1995) Eating well for older people. Report of an Expert Working Group. Further details from: 'Older People', Broadcast Support Services, PO Box 7, London W3 6XJ.

DOH (1992) The nutrition of elderly people. Report on Health and Social Subjects No 43. HMSO, London.

National Dairy Council (1992) Nutrition and Elderly People. Fact File No 9. The National Dairy Council, London.

Osteoporosis is a disorder characterised by a ↓ in bone mass, and results in fragile bones, causing fractures - it's predominantly a disease of middle life and old age & affects women > then men.

Section 5
Diet in Particular Situations

Chapter 19
Weight Control

That the attainment of ideal body weight makes an important contribution to health is undeniable and is one of the aims of healthy eating. Obesity is one of the most important health problems in the UK, but it should also be remembered that the process of 'dieting' is not without hazard.

Community pharmacists see the problems associated with weight control from two perspectives: first, through the sale of slimming products to individuals who may or may not need to lose weight, and secondly through the dispensing of prescriptions for disorders which may be related to the patient's obesity.

What is ideal weight?

Weight tables

Ideal weight has traditionally been defined by tables of 'desirable weight for height' published by life insurance companies. These tables are based on the mortality experience of people who have taken out life insurance policies, and they provide a range of weights for males and females of different heights.

Height should be measured without shoes, and weight without shoes and outdoor clothing. People who weigh more than 20% over the upper limit of weight for their height are considered to be obese.

Body mass index

Ideal weight may also be defined by using a calculation known as the Body Mass Index (BMI).

$$BMI = \frac{Weight \ (kg)}{Height \ (m)^2}$$

The desirable range is 20–25. Classification of BMI ranges is shown in Table 19.1. The person's height and weight may also be plotted on a chart (see Fig. 19.1).

Table 19.1   Classification of body mass index.

< 15	Severe emaciation
15–20	Underweight
20–25	Ideal weight
25–30	Overweight
30–40	Obese
> 40	Severe obesity

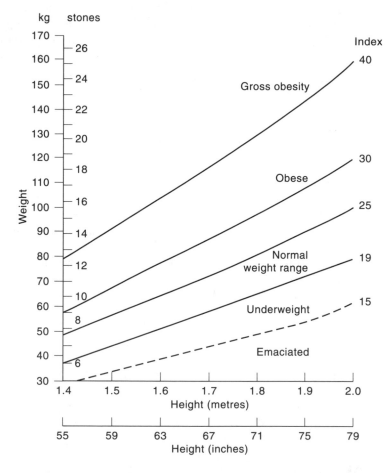

Fig. 19.1   Body Mass Index. Reproduced from *Eating Disorders. The Facts*. S. Abraham & D. Llewellyn-Jones, 1992, with kind permission of Oxford University Press, Oxford.

Waist/hip ratio

There is now evidence that the risk of metabolic disease (e.g. coronary heart disease, diabetes mellitus) is related to the distribution of fat as much, if not more, than the weight itself. Fat in and around the abdomen appears to increase the risk of disease, whereas fat deposited peripherally – in the arms and legs – does not.

Women tend to have more fat distributed peripherally, whereas men are likely to have more fat round the abdomen. This may be a contributing factor to the greater incidence of coronary heart disease in men.

Measurement of waist/hip ratio is becoming more common practice. The threshold value in men is 1.0 and in women 0.8. Above these values the risk of metabolic disease is high.

Prevalence of underweight, overweight and obesity

Underweight is relatively uncommon in the UK, and arises not from inadequate food supply but as a result of underlying physical or psychological disease. In the absence of physical disease a BMI of less than 15 is likely to be indicative of anorexia nervosa.

Obesity and overweight are increasing in the UK both in adults and in children. In 1980, 39% of adult males and 32% of adult females were overweight (BMI > 25), and obesity (BMI > 30) was present in 6% of adult men and 8% of adult women. By1996, 16% of men and 18% of women were obese, and a further 45% of men and 34% of women were overweight.

Causes of obesity

Human beings abide by the law of thermodynamics, so quite simply, obesity results from an excess of energy intake over expenditure. The most natural assumption is that fat people eat more than thin people or that fat people are lazy; this is not necessarily so. The only thing that is certain is that, at some time in their lives, overweight and obese people have eaten more than they needed, but there is little if any evidence to suggest that fat people are gluttons. While the link between excessive calorie intake and obesity is obvious, the idea that obesity is caused by gluttony is too simplistic. Since the 1950s, energy intake has actually fallen in the UK. As a nation, however, we have certainly become less active, and what seems to have happened is that, due to lack of physical activity, energy expenditure has fallen more than energy intake.

Overeating is a complex issue and one which is well beyond the scope of this book, but stress, boredom or feelings of lack of love are often suggested as psychological reasons for it. People eat for many reasons other than physiological hunger.

Obesity may be inherited. Whether this happens through transmission of family eating habits or genetic material is difficult to determine, but thin parents rarely produce fat children. In general, the fatter the parents the more likely it is that the children will also be fat. The discovery of an obesity gene raised the exciting possibility that obesity could be caused by a genetic mutation. The obesity gene is found in adipose tissue and encodes a protein called leptin. Leptin is secreted into the blood, and is thought, by means of negative feedback, to inform the brain about the size of the adipose tissue stores. A mutation in the obesity gene in mice, resulting in either insufficient or defective leptin can cause mice to become fat. Administration of leptin causes these mice to reduce their food intake. However, no such mutations have been found in the human obesity gene, and plasma levels of leptin are often elevated, rather than reduced, in obese people. Hopes that leptin may be useful clinically are therefore so far unfounded, but it may be that insights gained from its discovery could lead to useful drug treatments in the future.

Disease as a cause of obesity is quite rare and is certainly less common than obese people often like to believe. However, an underactive thyroid and some endocrine cancers may lead to excessive weight gain. Some drugs too may cause weight gain (see Chapter 26).

Health risks of obesity

Whether obesity is a disease or not is debatable, but the health hazards of obesity are well recognised. The life insurance industry has known from the beginning of the century that obese people are likely to die younger and are therefore less profitable to insure. Obesity (BMI > 30) is associated with the greatest disease risk, overweight (BMI 25–30) less so.

Cardiovascular disease, including hypertension, stroke and heart failure, occurs more often in people who are obese than in those who are not. Breathlessness on exertion is common in the obese, and there is an increased incidence of gastrointestinal problems such as hiatus hernia. Non-insulin dependent diabetes mellitus is relatively rare in people of normal weight, and arthritis tends to be exacerbated by weight gain. Obesity is also an important risk factor for gallstones and for sex hormone dependent cancers such as those of the breast, endometrium and prostate.

Obesity also leads to social discrimination in our society. The obese are often ridiculed and it is difficult to find fashionable clothes to fit.

Benefits of weight loss

Most of the health hazards of obesity are reversed by losing weight. However, the likelihood of gallstone formation may well increase during weight reduction in an obese person. This is because cholesterol from adipose tissue is mobilised, resulting in the bile becoming even more supersaturated with cholesterol. Once desirable weight is achieved the risk is reduced.

The psychological benefits are also important – feeling more active, increasing confidence and the ability to wear stylish clothes. But losing too much weight can be harmful, both physically and psychologically, and should not be pursued.

Management of weight loss

The only way to lose weight is to reduce the amount of energy obtained from the diet below the amount expended. The aim should be to lose weight gradually at the rate of about 1 kg a week. Every kilogram of adipose tissue represents about 29.4 MJ (7000 kcal), so a loss of 1 kg a week should be achieved when the daily energy intake is 4.2 MJ (1000 kcal) below output. In practice this usually means a diet providing 4.2 MJ (1000 kcal) for women and 6.3 MJ (1500 kcal) for men.

Weight loss programmes

A healthy weight loss programme does not mean 'dieting' in the sense described later on in this chapter. While 'dieting' may offer short-term benefits, it fails to encourage long-term changes in eating patterns which are essential if ideal body weight is to be maintained. There are no miraculous diets; sensible weight reduction involves eating a healthy diet of lower than normal energy content, and increasing exercise. Psychological factors producing motivation also need to be considered.

Healthy eating

Any weight reduction diet should be based on the principles of healthy eating (see Chapter 3). Although the diet must be lower in energy than the individual's normal diet, it is important that it should continue to provide adequate amounts of all the essential nutrients. A multivitamin supplement may be recommended if the diet provides less than 6.3 MJ (1500 kcal) a day. Emphasis should therefore be given to foods which are nutrient dense but low in energy. In practice this means reducing fat and sugar intake and increasing the intake of complex carbohydrates.

Fat is the richest source of energy in the diet providing 37.8 kJ/g (9 kcal/g) compared with carbohydrate and protein which both provide about 16.8 kJ/g (4 kcal/g). Foods high in fat should be replaced by lower fat alternatives, e.g. skimmed or semi-skimmed milk, reduced-fat spreads and cheeses. Meat should be lean, and poultry should be eaten without the skin. Fish consumption should be encouraged. Where beefburgers or sausages feature in the diet these should be low fat varieties. Chips should be eaten only occasionally; oven chips are lower in fat than fries. Frying should be discouraged or reduced to a minimum, and food baked, grilled or microwaved instead.

Sugar is a source of 'empty calories'. For the slimmer whose aim should be to eat a nutrient-dense but low energy diet this is an important point to remember. There is no point in eating sugary foods; they provide nothing but calories. People should be encouraged to give up sugar in drinks or use an artificial sweetener. Fizzy drinks and squashes should be of the 'diet' type. Chocolate, pastries, cakes and biscuits contain a lot of fat as well as sugar and should be eaten only occasionally.

Alcohol should not be forgotten as a source of calories; it provides 29.4 kJ/g (7 kcal/g) which is nearly as much energy as fat. A pint of beer provides 756 kJ (180 kcal) and a glass of wine 420 kJ (100 kcal). Alcohol should therefore be avoided, or at least restricted, on a weight-reducing diet.

Foods rich in starchy carbohydrates, particularly those rich in non-starch polysaccharides (NSP), should be encouraged. Wholegrain cereals, pulses and fruit and vegetables should form the main part of any weight-reducing diet. Raw fruit and vegetables are particularly useful as between-meal snacks.

The advice to eat bread and potatoes while trying to lose weight is a surprise to many. Carbohydrate has long been viewed as fattening and many slimmers avoid it. Yet on a weight-for-weight basis carbohydrate provides less than half the energy of fat. Bread and potatoes are not of themselves fattening; the problem lies in the fat that is put on them. Thus a slice of bread provides about 273 kJ (65 kcal); spreading with butter can easily double this figure. A portion of boiled potatoes provides 420 kJ (100 kcal); the same sized portion of chips provides 1.3 MJ (300 kcal).

It is not necessary to omit favourite foods completely. An occasional bar of chocolate or a packet of crisps does not ruin a diet. Believing that they do can induce such feelings of guilt in the slimmer that they abandon attempts to reduce weight altogether. Virtually any food can be included in moderation.

Exercise

Increasing exercise has many health benefits and should be encouraged, but in terms of producing an energy deficit the effect is not large. A man who goes jogging for an hour will use only 300 kcal more than he would have done sitting at his desk and to recommend this amount of exercise every day would not fit practically into many people's lifestyles. It would take a long time to reduce weight by exercise alone. Exercise is important in a weight loss programme but the energy content of the diet must also be reduced.

Psychological factors

Successful weight loss can only be achieved if a person wants to lose weight and is motivated to change eating habits. Advice should take account of current eating habits, lifestyle and background (see Chapter 1), and changes in food intake should be agreed with the person concerned.

Some general advice which can be given in addition to dietary advice includes:

- Eating from a smaller plate
- Keeping as busy as possible
- Avoiding shopping when hungry

- Making a shopping list and sticking to it
- Eating slowly and chewing well
- Avoiding periods of starvation

Support is often a vital ingredient in successful weight loss, and people can be encouraged to return to the pharmacy for discussion of their progress. A weighing machine provides a focal point for dialogue and weight monitoring.

Special diets

The diet industry has increased dramatically in recent years and there are currently in print more than 200 books on the subject of diet and slimming for the general reader. There are also several slimming magazines and many others which carry articles about dieting.

Discussion of individual diets is beyond the scope of this book, but if pharmacists are asked about any one in particular they should compare it with the principles of healthy eating. Many special diets are nutritionally unsound, particularly if they rely on one or very few foods (e.g. the grapefruit diet), which can easily result in nutrient deficiency if pursued for more than a few days.

Drastic or 'crash' diets where energy intake is dramatically reduced should be discouraged for a number of reasons. First, any diet that provides less than 4.2 MJ (100 kcal) a day is likely to be lacking in nutrients; second, it is likely to be unpalatable and antisocial and difficult to stick to for more than a few days; and thirdly it may result in the loss of lean tissue.

If lean tissue is lost, basal metabolic rate (BMR) falls and as a consequence the body's ability to use energy also falls. When a person starts to eat normally again, weight can only be maintained on a lower energy intake than before the 'diet' was started; hence the suggestion that 'dieting makes you fat'.

The value of special diets to some slimmers lies in their structured approach. To be given a set of rigid menus – at least for a few days or weeks – is a relief to many slimmers. The problem is that when the diet is abandoned old habits are taken up again, and any weight that has been lost is quickly regained. Special diets do nothing to encourage change in eating habits which will be necessary if ideal weight is to be maintained in the long term.

Slimming clubs

The value of joining a slimming club lies in the support it can give. Being with other people who are trying to achieve the same ends can do much to reduce the sense of isolation felt by many slimmers.

Care should be taken to choose a reputable slimming club. Some GP practices are setting up discussion groups for patients who need to lose weight, and these will normally be run by a practice nurse or dietitian. Pharmacists should find out if such groups operate in their area and refer people who need to lose weight.

Slimming products

There are several types of slimming products, many of which are available in pharmacies:

- Very low calorie diets (VLCDs)
- Meal replacement products
- Reduced-fat or reduced-energy products
- Sugar substitutes
- Calorie counted meals
- OTC appetite suppressants
- Herbal products

A slimming claim, e.g. 'Can help slimming or weight control only as part of a calorie (or energy) controlled diet', can only be used if the food will contribute to weight loss.

Very low calorie diets (VLCDs)

The term 'very low calorie diet' is taken to mean a commercially prepared diet which reduces the energy intake below 2.5 MJ (600 kcal)/day for several consecutive days or weeks by total substitution of normal meals. It does not include preparations or regimens which seek to achieve similar low energy intakes by partial replacement only (i.e. by replacing one or more meals with a low calorie substitute while leaving the rest of the dietary pattern unchanged), or by overall reduction in normal food intake. Some of these diets are available through special counsellors (e.g. the Cambridge Diet). Each day's supply provides sufficient nutrients including protein, vitamins, minerals and trace elements.

VLCDs may be useful in obese people who have tried conventional methods and failed, but they should ideally be used only after medical referral. They should not be used for longer than a month, and it is important that plenty of fluid is drunk (at least three or four pints a day).

VLCDs are not suitable for the following groups of people:

- Patients with cardiovascular disorders, severe hepatic or renal disease, gout and porphyria
- Individuals with psychological states such as schizophrenia, eating disorders and other severe behavioural disorders, and severe depression
- Individuals on lithium therapy
- Patients with diabetes mellitus on insulin or oral hypoglycaemics, who without adjustment of dosage may be at risk of hypoglycaemia
- Patients on antihypertensives, who without reduction in dosage may be at risk of hypotensive episodes
- Infants, children, pregnant and breast-feeding women and the elderly

Meal replacement products

Meal replacements are intended to replace one or at the most two meals a day in combination with one or two conventional meals. They generally provide between 420 and 1050 kJ (100–250 kcal) a meal and include drinks, biscuits and soups. Each meal generally provides around one-third of the body's requirement for vitamins and minerals. Some people find meal replacements convenient as a means of counting calories, particularly when at work, but conventional foods tend to be cheaper, can be just as nutritious and are more likely to help to change eating habits.

Reduced fat or reduced energy products

The market for reduced fat and low energy products has increased dramatically and there is a wide range available including reduced fat milks, spreads, cheeses, mayonnaise, sausages, beefburgers, ice cream, crisps and low calorie soft and fizzy drinks. These can be useful in reducing the energy content of the diet without substantially changing the character of the diet.

Diabetic foods are not suitable for weight reduction. Although they are often sugar free, they may be as high in energy as their non-diabetic counterparts.

Sugar substitutes

There are two types of sugar substitutes: those which supply no or almost no energy (non-nutritive sweeteners), and those which supply energy (nutritive sweeteners). Non-nutritive sweeteners available in the UK include saccharin, aspartame and acesulfame K (see Table 19.2). The chief nutritive sweetener used is sorbitol and this is mainly used in diabetic foods.

Non-nutritive sweeteners can play a part in reducing energy intake, but the eventual aim should be to eat fewer sweet-tasting foods. Artificial sweeteners are thought to be safe in normal intakes, e.g. the amount used in three or four cups of tea a day, but excessive use should be avoided. Saccharin has been associated with bladder cancer in rats, but is generally thought to be safe in humans. Patients with phenylketonuria should avoid aspartame and foods and medicines which contain it (see Chapter 9). Aspartame does not leave the bitter aftertaste which is often associated with saccharin.

Calorie counted meals

These are complete meals – often frozen – providing around 1.3 MJ (300 kcal)/meal. These products are convenient in that they 'count calories' and decide the size of the meal, but they are expensive.

OTC products

These basically fall into two categories – appetite suppressants and products

Table 19.2 Sugar substitutes.

Brand name	Manufacturer	Sweetener
Canderel	Monsanto	
Spoonful		Aspartame
tablets		Aspartame
Flix	Monsanto	
tablets		Aspartame
Hermesetas	Jenks Group	
Gold		
granulated		Aspartame
tablets		Aspartame
Original		
liquid		Saccharin
tablets		Saccharin
Natrena	Douwe Egberts	
tablets		Saccharin
Sucron	Roche Consumer Health	
powder		Sucrose and saccharin
Sweet 'n' low	Santo Products	
minicubes		Saccharin
powder		Saccharin
tablets		Saccharin
Sweetex	Crookes Healthcare	
granulated		Aspartame and saccharin
solution		Saccharin
tablets		Saccharin

which reduce fat absorption. Appetite suppressants are usually in the form of tablets or powders, and are designed to be taken before meals with a drink to make people feel less hungry and therefore eat less at a meal. They are ineffective in the long term, but may have a short-term placebo effect.

Some are based on bulking agents such as bran or methylcellulose (e.g. Bran Slim) and induce a sense of fullness by swelling in the stomach. Care should always be taken to swallow these products with plenty of fluid because there is a risk of obstructing the gut. Others contain sugar (e.g. Slim Disks) and reduce hunger by raising the blood glucose.

Chitosan, present in Fat Magnets and Chilo-Slimmer tablets, is claimed to reduce weight by increasing faecal fat excretion. Anecdotally, it seems to work for some people, but there have been no large-scale clinical trials investigating its efficacy and long-term safety.

Herbal products

There are a number of herbal slimming products available. Some are intended to reduce weight by a laxative effect and some by a diuretic action. Although they may induce weight loss in the short term, they have no effect on body fat.

Drugs

The place of drugs in the treatment of obesity is the subject of a great deal of debate. A number of drugs have been advocated over the years for the treatment of obesity, but their use has been controversial. This has been partly out of concern about side-effects; and two anti-obesity drugs – fenfluramine and dexfenfluramine – have recently been withdrawn for this reason.

However, a report from the Royal College of Physicians in 1998 recommended that, in the light of the alarming rise in obesity, drugs may be justified, particularly for those who are obese, and also for those who are overweight with other conditions, such as diabetes. However, drugs should only be considered when dietary and lifestyle modifications have failed to work. The only drugs currently licensed in the UK are orlistat, methylcellulose and phentermine, although several others are in the pipeline.

Bulk forming drugs

Bulk forming drugs used in obesity include methylcellulose and sterculia. When administered with a drink they swell in the stomach and create a sensation of satiety. Taken just before a meal they may help to reduce energy intake.

Surgery

Surgical techniques may occasionally be used to reduce food intake in obese people. Wiring of the jaws prevents intake of solid food and the patient drinks through a straw. The size of the stomach can be reduced by gastric stapling and absorption of food by jejunal bypass surgery. Such techniques are not without hazard and are only used as a last resort.

Dieting

Although many people in the UK are overweight or obese, many more believe themselves to be overweight. Concern about weight and shape has become an obsession in Western culture particularly among women, and there is some evidence that it is starting to increase in Asia and Africa too. At least twice as many women may be attempting to lose weight as is necessary for health.

Constant dieting can easily become a way of life. As many as 15% of women in the UK may be chaotic eaters with an unpredictable collection of eating and weight loss behaviours, which, although culturally acceptable, may eventually lead to more definable eating disorders.

In contrast to a hundred years ago when it was fashionable for women to be fat, the slim woman today is seen as attractive, healthy, happy, fit and popular. Although the fashion for extreme thinness may disappear – and there is evidence that this is starting to happen – the most stylish clothes still tend to be designed for slim figures. Successful slimming tends to increase self-esteem and produces a sense of achievement.

This is all very well if weight really needs to be reduced, but the obsession with weight loss has become something of a health hazard; the cost of slimming can be extremely high. Dieting may involve control to such an unnatural degree that the slimmer suffers from chronic stress. The anxiety caused by restrained eating is likely to lead to overeating and a cycle of weight loss and weight gain such that over a period of time there may be no net weight loss at all.

The hazards of dieting may therefore outweigh the hazards of obesity. This is not to endorse overeating nor to suggest that obesity should not be treated, but weight loss should only be embarked upon where it is really necessary and should involve only moderate restriction based on healthy eating guidelines.

Eating disorders

The eating disorders anorexia nervosa and bulimia nervosa are distressing conditions which predominantly affect adolescent and young adult women, although increasingly men and older women may suffer. Patients are often intelligent and from middle-class families. Eating disorders have a strong psychological component, and patients often have problems with family and interpersonal relationships, perfections, self-esteem, obsessional behaviour and high levels of anxiety and depression. They often occur as a result of efforts to diet during the teenage years.

Anorexia nervosa

The word anorexia means loss of appetite, but most people with anorexia do not actually lose their appetite. They simply deny hunger and have an intense fear of food and becoming fat. Excessive exercise may be used as a means of preventing weight gain. The hallmark of anorexia is profound weight loss, and the prevalence in the UK is about 1%. A number of other symptoms are commonly associated with anorexia, including constipation, amenorrhoea and intolerance to cold. As weight loss progresses, hypotension, bradycardia and hypothermia may be seen. The skin becomes dry and scaly. Anorexia can be fatal.

Bulimia

Bulimia means abnormal hunger and has become commonly known as 'binge eating'. It is characterised by the ingestion of large quantities of food over a short period of time, which may be followed by induced vomiting. Laxative abuse is also common and pharmacists will be aware of this. Menstruation may be irregular.

Energy intake can be as high as 210 MJ (50 000 kcal) during a binge, and although most people with bulimia prefer foods that are rich in carbohydrates any kind of food may be chosen. Secrecy about eating is common in bulimia, and bingeing usually takes place at home and alone. Weight may well be normal; most people with bulimia have a morbid fear of becoming fat. Weight is controlled by alternating bingeing with periods of starvation.

The pharmacist's role

Treatment of eating disorders is complex, and counselling is well beyond the scope of the pharmacist. Still, by being aware of the symptoms, pharmacists can encourage medical referral and make a contribution to the early recognition of such disorders. Pharmacists may also have a role in supporting both patients and their parents.

Further reading

British Nutrition Foundation (1999) *Obesity. The Report of the British Nutrition Foundation Task Force.* Blackwell Science, Oxford.

DoH (1987) The use of very low calorie diets in obesity. Report on Health and Social Subjects No 31. HMSO, London.

DoH (1995) Reversing the increasing problem of obesity in England. A report from the Nutrition and Physical Activity Task Forces. Available from the Department of Health, PO Box 410, Wetherby, LS23 7LN.

The Health Education Authority (1991) *Obesity and Overweight.* The Health Education Authority, London.

Royal College of Physicians (1998) *Clinical Management of Overweight and Obese Patients.* The Royal College of Physicians, London.

Useful addresses

Anorexics Anonymous. Tel: 0208 748 3994.

Eating Disorders Association, Sackville Place, 44 Magdalen Street, Norwich NR3 1JU. Tel: 01603 621414.

Overeaters Anonymous for London and South-East, c/o Manor Gardens Centre, 6–9 Manor Gardens, London N7 6LA; for rest of England and Wales, PO Box 19, Stretford, Manchester M32 9EB. Tel: 0208 442 0214.

Weight Watchers (UK), Kidwells Park House, Kidwells Park Drive, Maidenhead, Berks SL6 8YT. Tel: 0345 123000.

Chapter 20
Sports and Athletics

There are many misconceptions about the role of nutrition in sports, and many supplements are promoted to improve performance. The main consideration for the athlete is the provision of sufficient energy.

Energy metabolism

The main sources of energy for working muscles are shown in Fig. 20.1. Energy is obtained most efficiently and quickly from glucose, which can be obtained either from the stores of glycogen in the liver and muscle or to a

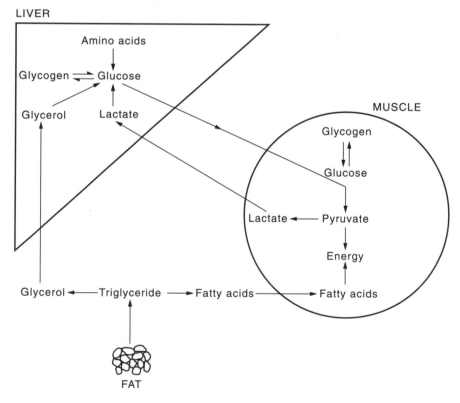

Fig. 20.1   Major sources of energy for the muscles.

lesser extent from amino acids. Stores of energy in the form of glucose are not large compared with needs; even in a trained athlete, they can provide no more than about 3.4 MJ (800 kcal) which could easily be used up in an hour's intensive activity.

During endurance events the body therefore needs an alternative source of energy. This is provided by fat. Stores of fat are far greater than those of glucose and the potential energy yield from fatty acid oxidation is enormous. The rate of energy production from fat, however, is relatively slow compared with that from glucose, making fat a much less efficient source of energy. Exercising muscles therefore obtain energy from a mixture of fat and glucose, and the proportions used depend on the intensity and duration of the activity.

At rest or at low exercise intensity the rate of energy production is not too critical, and fat provides most of the energy with glucose supplying a smaller proportion.

During more intensive activity the body needs energy faster, and about two-thirds are provided by glucose and one-third by fat. Activities such as sprinting demand such a rapid energy supply that normal aerobic conversion of glucose is too slow. Energy can be provided more rapidly by the anaerobic conversion of glucose to lactate, but build-up of lactate in the muscle causes fatigue, so this process cannot continue indefinitely. Nevertheless, anaerobic respiration is essential during short bouts of intensive activity.

As exercise continues, particularly during endurance events, the glycogen stores decline and must be conserved. Fatty acids again become a major source of energy, and glucose may be obtained not only from glycogen but also from amino acids and glycerol (produced by the breakdown of triglyceride – see Figure 20.1).

During any exercise the aim is to conserve glycogen. It is interesting that well trained athletes tend to adapt and oxidise more fat than glucose, but whenever exercise is performed some glycogen will also be used. And glycogen can only be obtained from carbohydrate. The longer and more intense the exercise the greater is the need for carbohydrate.

Nutritional requirements

The principles of nutrition are no different for athletes than for non-athletes and dietary advice should be based on healthy eating guidelines (see Chapter 3). There are no miracle diets. The overall quality of the diet is just as important as the food and drink consumed before, during and after an event.

Carbohydrate

The importance of carbohydrate cannot be overemphasised. Just as for non-athletes, carbohydrate should provide 50–55% of the dietary energy. For an athlete consuming a high energy diet (eg 16.8 MJ or 400 kcal/day) this is an enormous quantity of carbohydrate (500 g). It could be obtained, for example, by consuming two large bowls of muesli, six slices of bread, a large portion of rice or pasta and a large baked potato.

Many athletes obtain a large proportion of their carbohydrate from sugary foods because they are convenient. Starchy foods (e.g. bread, potatoes, pasta, rice and cereals) are a healthier choice and should be encouraged. Sugar intake should be reduced but this is not quite as important for athletes as for non-athletes: if sugar intake is reduced and not replaced with starchy foods the all-important glycogen stores will not be replaced. Sugary foods need not be excluded from an athlete's diet.

To eat a diet rich in complex carbohydrate which provides sufficient energy for the athlete requires careful organisation. Many athletes train straight after work and allow little time for buying, cooking and eating food. Ease and speed of food preparation are important and athletes often rely on fast food and take-aways. If this is the case, baked potatoes, muesli bars and pizzas are the healthiest choices.

Carbohydrate loading

Unlike many nutritional practices favoured by athletes, this does have some scientific basis. Starting about a week before the sporting event, it involves eating a low carbohydrate diet for 3 days followed by a high carbohydrate diet for 3 days, and its aim is to increase the glycogen stores. Care should be taken not to overdo the days of carbohydrate restriction. Even after 3 days of carbohydrate-rich diet, many athletes approach an event with low glycogen stores. Diabetics should not use this technique without medical referral.

If handled properly, carbohydrate loading can be beneficial, particularly for endurance events lasting for longer than 2 hours, but not for those lasting less than 60 minutes. Because glycogen is stored with water, carbohydrate loading can reduce the risk of dehydration. Accumulation of water does however lead to weight gain, and this can be a disadvantage in sports which require specific weight ranges, e.g. for jockeys. It is ineffective if repeated more than two or three times a year.

Protein

Intensive training results in deposition of protein in the muscle which leads to an increased requirement for protein. In most cases adequate protein can be obtained from the diet. Eating large quantities of meat, milk, eggs and cheese is expensive, and because it may reduce the appetite for carbohydrate-rich foods it should not be encouraged. Athletes who are concerned about protein should be referred to a sports nutritionist or dietitian.

Fluid and electrolytes

Prolonged exercise leads to a loss of water and electrolytes from the body. As much as 2 litres of fluid an hour can be lost during prolonged exercise in a hot environment.

Thirst is not always a reliable indicator of the state of hydration, and athletes should always drink plenty of fluid before, during and after an event. Large quantities of fluid at once should be avoided because of the risk of nausea and stomach cramp. Cold fluid leaves the stomach faster than warm fluid so drinks should be consumed at a temperature of 8–13°C. Athletes should be advised to drink 200–500 ml of fluid about 20 minutes before the event. Urine production falls as soon as exercise begins, so there should be no necessity for a toilet stop. Regular stops for fluid are essential during an endurance event.

The need for electrolytes during an event is not so great except perhaps for sodium in events lasting longer than 4 hours in a hot climate. Sodium can normally be replaced by sprinkling salt on the food after the activity.

Sports supplements

Sports supplements can be broadly divided into the following groups:

- Energy supplements
- Sports drinks
- Amino acid supplements
- Vitamins and minerals
- Caffeine
- Lactic acid buffers
- Herbs

Energy supplements

Adequate energy should ideally be provided from normal food, but it has already been said that athletes may devote little time to food preparation. In addition, some athletes cannot face conventional food on the day of an event because of nausea or nervousness or both.

Meal replacement drinks, including those marketed for slimming (e.g. Slim Fast and Slender) and convalescence (e.g. Build Up and Complan) as well as those for sports, may be used by athletes who for whatever reason are unable to eat enough food.

Sports drinks

There are two types of sports drinks. These are fluid replacement drinks and carbohydrate replacement drinks.

Fluid replacement drinks

The importance of fluid during exercise has already been stressed. Fluid absorption should be maximised, and one of the factors influencing the movement of fluid into the body is the osmolality of the drink. If the drink is hypotonic with respect to the body fluids, water will move from the gut into the body. On the other hand, if the drink is hypertonic, water will be secreted rather than absorbed.

Small amounts of glucose and electrolytes help to maximise fluid intake, but if the concentration of these substances is greatly increased as in carbo-hydrate replacement drinks (see next section), fluid absorption is compromised. The value of electrolytes in fluid replacement drinks is in the promotion of fluid absorption, not the supply of electrolytes.

The optimal concentration of carbohydrate in a fluid replacement drink is about 5–7%. Products exceeding these concentrations should be avoided or diluted where fluid replacement is the main aim (see Table 10.2). Fruit juices, for example, should be diluted to half strength.

Table 20.1 Carbohydrate content[1] of proprietary drinks (ready to drink where purchased as a concentrate).

Drink	Percentage carbohydrate
Hydra-Fuel (Twinlab)	7
Isostar (Wander)	7
Lucozade (SmithKline Beecham)	19
Lucozade Light (SmithKline Beecham)	5
Lucozade Sport (SmithKline Beecham)	7
Lucozade Sport low calorie (SmithKline Beecham)	0.5
Ribena (SmithKline Beecham)	15
Ribena low sugar (SmithKline Beecham)	5
Robinson's barley waters (Colman's of Norwich)	5
Fruit squashes – average	5
High juice fruit squashes – average	8
Diet fruit squashes – average	0.5
Fruit juices – average	10
Fruit juice drinks – average	10

[1] Ideal carbohydrate content for fluid replacement is 5–7%.

Carbohydrate replacement drinks

Carbohydrate replacement drinks contain more carbohydrate than fluid replacement drinks – normally about 100 g a serving, providing a concentration of 20% when water is added. Increasing glucose concentration results in a solution of high osmolality, which not only reduces fluid absorption but may also produce an osmotic diarrhoea. A better source of carbohydrate is glucose polymer such as maltodextrin, which on a weight-for-weight basis provides the same energy as glucose but with a lower osmolality. This enables glucose to be delivered to the bloodstream more rapidly. It is for this reason that many sports drinks contain maltodextrin.

Carbohydrate replacement drinks and any other carbohydrate-rich products, such as glucose sweets, should be avoided within the 30 minutes before an event because they increase blood glucose levels resulting in increased insulin secretion. Secretion of insulin causes blood glucose levels to fall rapidly and inhibits fat mobilisation. This results in a greater reliance on glycogen stores, and fatigue sets in more rapidly.

Excessive amounts of these products should also be avoided during exercise. Carbohydrate is of no benefit unless the event is a long one, and in that case it is better to consume small amounts every half hour. The most appropriate use of carbohydrate replacement drinks is after the activity as part of the refuelling process. They may be used in addition to starchy foods.

Amino acid supplements

It is a common belief among athletes that amino acid supplements increase muscle mass, but there is little evidence for this. Some supplements contain branched chain amino acids (leucine, isoleucine and valine) because it has been suggested that these are taken up by active muscle during exercise, while most of the other amino acids are released.

Vitamins and minerals

Some vitamins and minerals are involved in energy production, and requirements do increase with energy expenditure, but if energy intake increases, the intake of vitamins and minerals is likely to increase too. This is one reason why it is better to increase energy intake with complex carbohydrates rather than sugar; sugar provides nothing but calories.

Iron deficiency is a possibility in athletes, leading to so-called 'sports anaemia'. This may arise as a result of exercise stress, which leads to increased destruction of red blood cells, or it may be a consequence of the natural increase in blood volume which occurs in many trained athletes. Sports anaemia is a particular risk in endurance runners of both sexes, and in all female athletes particularly if they have heavy periods. A mild iron product (providing around 20 mg of iron) should be recommended.

The only other circumstances in which vitamin and mineral supplements are justified are where the diet is poor, or where weight reduction is being pursued because of competing in sports where specific weight categories are important. These include rowing, horse racing, combat sports, running and gymnastics.

Caffeine

Caffeine has often been used by athletes because it promotes fat mobilisation and spares glycogen, but several cups of black coffee or cola drinks are needed to produce this effect. Caffeine is also found in some OTC medicines (e.g. some pain killers and cold remedies).

Large amounts of caffeine are banned by the International Olympic Committee. One or two cups of coffee is not excessive, but several cups could increase urine levels of caffeine beyond the permitted limit of 12 µg/ml.

Lactic acid buffers

During intensive exercise such as sprinting, the muscles produce energy anaerobically, leading to the build-up of lactic acid and muscle fatigue. Bicarbonate solutions are promoted as a means of mopping up the excess lactic acid thereby reducing the risk of fatigue. Whether they work or not is debatable; if the exercise lasts less than 2 minutes, they are unlikely to work because there is insufficient time to remove lactic acid from the muscle. With exercise that lasts longer (e.g. 2–15 minutes), they may work because there is more time to mop up the excess lactate. Bicarbonate may cause nausea and diarrhoea, and any possible benefits may not be worth the side-effects.

Herbs

A variety of herbs and plant ingredients is used in sports supplements. These include ginseng, guarana, kola nut, kelp and alfalfa. There is little evidence that these substances have any beneficial effect on performance.

The dietary advice discussed in this chapter is summarised below:

Dietary advice for athletes.

(1) The diet should be based on healthy eating guidelines
(2) The importance of carbohydrate – particularly starchy carbohydrate – should be emphasised
(3) A meal should be eaten 3 hours before exercise rather than just before it
(4) Glucose should be avoided in the half hour before the event
(5) A drink of 200–500 ml should be consumed 20 minutes before the event
(6) The importance of regular fluid stops should be stressed
(7) During endurance events carbohydrate should be replenished every half an hour with starchy foods, confectionery, glucose or a glucose polymer fluid
(8) After the exercise, carbohydrate and fluid replenishment should start immediately
(9) All food and drink consumed during a sports event should be tested for individual suitability during training

---

Further reading

Brouns, F. (1993) *Nutritional Needs of Athletes*. John Wiley and Sons Ltd, Chichester.

Pearce, J. (1990) *Eat to Compete*. Reed Books, New Zealand. (Available from the Pharmaceutical Press, PO Box 11640, Wellington, New Zealand.)

Wooton, S. (1989) *Nutrition for Sport*. Simon and Schuster, London.

Useful addresses

Sports Nutrition Foundation, c/o London Sports Medicine Institute, Medical College of St Bartholomew's Hospital, Charterhouse Sq, London EC1M 6BQ. Tel: 0207 250 0493.

Chapter 21
Vegetarianism

The new wave of interest in health and animal rights has encouraged increasing numbers of individuals to reject meat. Some cultural minorities in the UK also adopt vegetarian diets for religious reasons (see Chapter 23).

No longer relegated to the fringes of society, vegetarianism has become much more accepted particularly amongst the young. For many it does not just mean a change of diet but a new way of life. It is associated with environmental and 'green' issues and to some extent with the 'health food' movement. Most vegetarians are concerned about health and nutrition, and proportionately fewer of them smoke and drink alcohol than is the case for non-vegetarians.

Whether vegetarians are any healthier than omnivores is questionable. Even if they are, it is not necessarily due to the diet. Vegetarians differ from omnivores in many aspects of lifestyle other than rejection of meat. Use of prescription and OTC medicines tends to be lower in vegetarians than in non-vegetarians, but the incidence of minor health problems such as colds and sore throats is not.

A vegetarian diet may be protective against the development of a range of diseases, including coronary heart disease, some cancers, diabetes mellitus, obesity, constipation and hypertension, but the link between vegetarianism and disease needs further investigation.

What is vegetarianism?

Vegetarianism defies specific definition. The Vegetarian Society defines a vegetarian diet as one that includes grains, pulses, nuts, seeds, fruit and vegetables, and excludes all meat, poultry, game, fish and their derivatives, with or without the use of free-range eggs, milk and dairy products. Within this broad definition a whole range of diets are practised with varying degrees of exclusion (see Table 21.1).

The first stage in becoming a vegetarian is usually to give up red meat, and this may be followed by exclusion of poultry and fish. Some vegetarians object to battery or intensively farmed eggs because they believe that the method of production is cruel; others object to cow's milk for similar reasons. Some also avoid certain food ingredients and additives (see Table 21.1).

Table 21.1 Classification of vegetarian diets.

Type	Diet
Demi- or semi-vegetarian	Excludes all red meat or all meat; poultry may be excluded; fish is included
Lacto-ovovegetarian	Excludes all meat, poultry and fish; milk, dairy products and eggs are consumed
Lacto-vegetarian	Excludes all meat, poultry, fish and eggs; milk and dairy products consumed
Vegan	Excludes all food of animal origin including foods processed with animal products, and sometimes honey; includes pulses, cereals, nuts, seeds, fruit, vegetables and vegetable oils
Fruitarian	An extreme form of veganism which forbids killing plants; excludes pulses and cereals as well as all food of animal origin; includes raw and dried fruit, nuts, honey and olive oil.
Macrobiotic	An extreme diet followed by adherents of the Taoist philosophy, which states that bodily and spiritual health is dependent on the forces of Yin (negative) and Yang (positive); the diet moves through progressively restrictive levels until only brown rice is consumed

Note: As well as the more obvious ingredients such as lard and suet, the following food ingre dients may also be unacceptable to some vegetarians: albumen, aspic, cochineal, collagen, gelatin, isinglass, lactose, lecithin, rennet and whey (for more details refer to the *Vegetarian Handbook* produced by the Vegetarian Society); and additives E120, E631, E635, E904 and E920 (see Chapter 4).

Individuals may move through different stages of vegetarianism, excluding different foods and ingredients, eventually giving up all animal products to become vegans. Some experiment with vegetarianism and then later retreat from it. What will be avoided or consumed at any one time will therefore be impossible to tell. There is no such thing as a typical vegetarian; before giving advice questions should always be asked about the nature of the diet.

How many vegetarians?

The 1999 Realeat Survey indicated that 5% of the adult population (aged 16 years and over) were vegetarians, and that in addition 8.6% were avoiding red meat. This combined group represents 14% of the population and 7.5 million people. Numbers have trebled since 1984. In addition more than 10% of children and teenagers are vegetarian or avoiding red meat, and 43% of adults are trying to reduce red meat consumption, a practice which has been encouraged by the BSE scare.

Vegetarian nutrition

A well planned vegetarian diet can be a healthy diet but it can also be a badly balanced one. Vegetables on their own, for example, do not constitute a balanced meal.

Energy

Most vegetarian diets provide sufficient energy for adults but care should be taken with infants and children. Vegetarian diets tend to be bulky, and whilst such a diet is fine for sedentary adults who do not need to gain weight it may provide too little energy for a growing chid. If infants are weaned on to a vegetarian diet, care should be taken to include energy-dense foods such as pulses, grains and nut butters, rather than relying exclusively on bulky vegetables and fruit.

Protein

It is a common misconception that vegetarian diets are deficient in protein. More than enough protein can easily be obtained without eating meat, milk, cheese or eggs.

Protein is a source of amino acids. There are essential amino acids, which must be supplied in the diet; and non-essential amino acids, which can be synthesised in the body. Traditionally, animal foods have been considered to be first class proteins, because they supply all the essential amino acids, and plant foods as second class proteins because they are generally lacking in one or more essential amino acids.

However, if different plant foods are eaten together, the amino acids will complement each other. What is lacking in one food will be compensated for by another. Cereals for example are lacking in lysine but contain adequate cystine and methionine. Pulses and nuts contain adequate lysine but are deficient in cystine and methionine. Other complementary combinations are illustrated in Fig. 21.1.

Vegans have traditionally been advised to combine plant proteins at every meal. This is no longer considered essential. However, the guideline is a useful educational tool, since it is important to include a wide variety of plant proteins throughout the day.

Fat

Vegetarian diets are not necessarily lower in fat than omnivorous diets. Cheese contains far more fat than lean meat so a vegetarian diet could contain more fat than an ordinary mixed diet. Mixed dishes containing pulses, rice and pasta are likely to be lower in fat unless they are fried or eaten with fatty sauces.

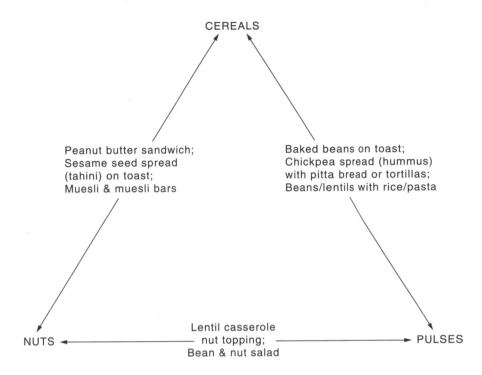

Fig. 21.1 Complementary combinations of vegetable proteins.

Vitamins

A well planned vegetarian diet can provide an adequate intake of vitamins, but the more restrictive the diet the greater the risk of deficiency. Some women pursue vegetarian diets and reduce their energy intake at the same time; this exposes them to an increased risk of nutrient deficiency.

Vegans may be deficient in vitamins B_{12} and D. Vitamin deficiency is also a possibility in new vegetarians whose absorption mechanisms may take a few months to adapt to the different diet.

Vitamin B_{12}

Vitamin B_{12} is found almost exclusively in animal products, so vegan diets are the ones most likely to be lacking in the vitamin. Vegetarians who include at least half a pint of milk or 50 g of cheese a day in their diet are less likely to suffer deficiency.

Vitamin B_{12} is stored in the liver, and in people who have previously eaten meat, stores can last 3–4 years before deficiency develops. Symptoms of vitamin B_{12} deficiency include megaloblastic anaemia, neuropathy, and infertility in females. Other less specific symptoms include sore tongue, weakness, tingling and numbness of the fingers and toes, and gastrointestinal problems.

Vegans must supplement the diet with vitamin B_{12} – preferably by consuming fortified foods (see Table 21.2) or by taking a dietary supplement. The Reference Nutrient Intake (RNI) is 1.5 µg/day. This can be obtained from half a pint of fortified soya milk.

Table 21.2 Examples of vegetarian and vegan sources of vitamin B_{12}.

Food	Vitamin B_{12}/portion (µg)
Dairy foods	
Cow's milk: half a pint	0.8
Yoghurt: 150 g	0.3
Cheese, Cheddar: 50 g	0.4
Egg: 1 large	0.4
Vegan foods	
Margarines	
Pure margarine: 10 g (Mathews Foods)	0.5
Seaweed: Laverbread (100 g)	1.6
Soya milk	
Gold: half a pint (Unisoy)	1.5
Plamil: half a pint, diluted (Plamil)	3.2
Vegetable protein mixes	
Burgamix: 100 g (Protoveg)	3.6
Sosmix: 100 g (Protoveg)	1.8
Yeast extracts	
Marmite: 5 g (CPC)	0.4
Natex: 5 g (Modern Health Products)	0.4
Vecon: 5 g (Modern Health Products)	0.6

Increasingly, manufacturers are adding vitamin B_{12} to their products, e.g. breakfast cereals and soft drinks such as Ribena, but these may be unacceptable to vegans because they contain animal residues or too much sugar or both. The belief that fermented soya products such as tempeh contain the vitamin has been proven to be unfounded. Boiling milk also destroys the vitamin.

Vitamin D

Vitamin D is obtained normally by the action of sunlight on the skin, and dietary sources are less important for most people.

The exceptions are children, pregnant and breast-feeding women and Asians, many of whom are vegetarians. Those who consume milk and dairy products will obtain some vitamin D, but vegans can only obtain it by eating fortified foods. Whilst some fortified foods are acceptable to vegans, several (e.g. most breakfast cereals) are not. Foods fortified with vitamin D_2 are acceptable but many are fortified with vitamin D_3 which is obtained from animals.

Minerals

Iron

Meat is a rich source of iron so vegetarians may be at slighter risk of anaemia than omnivores. Vegans often have higher intakes of iron then people consuming ordinary diets, but it must be remembered that iron from plant foods is not so well absorbed as iron from animal sources.

Vitamin C promotes the absorption of iron from plant foods, so all vegetarians should be encouraged to consume a rich source of vitamin C (e.g. citrus fruit or juice, green vegetables, raw salad) at every meal. Tannins (found in tea) reduce iron absorption from plant foods, so tea is best drunk between meals rather than with them. Iron-rich plant foods should also be emphasised (see Appendix 3).

Calcium

Calcium intake in lacto-vegetarians is usually adequate but is likely to be low in vegans. Low calcium intake does not necessarily lead to deficiency, because the body can adapt by increasing absorption, but it is important to emphasise the value of calcium-rich plant foods (see Appendix 4). White bread is a significant source of calcium for those who eat it, but many vegetarians eat wholemeal bread which is not fortified. Vegetarians who make their own bread can increase their calcium intake by adding 1 level teaspoon of calcium carbonate BP to each 500-g bag of wholemeal flour; four thick slices of such bread will supply about 500 mg of calcium.

Zinc

Vegan diets may be deficient in zinc because foods considered to be the best sources (e.g. meat, milk, cheese and eggs) are excluded. Vegetarian diets are often high in non-starch polysaccharides (NSP) and phytate, both of which have been thought to prejudice the absorption of zinc and other minerals. However, there is little evidence of poor zinc status in long-term vegetarians; if intake is low, it is likely that the body adapts by increasing absorption.

Iodine

The main sources of iodine in the UK diet are milk and dairy products, and it is therefore not surprising that vegans often have very low intakes. The RNI for iodine is 140 µg/day. This amount could easily be provided by iodised salt but the use of excessive quantities should be discouraged for two reasons: first, a healthy diet should not contain large amounts of salt, and, secondly, uncontrolled amounts of iodine may upset thyroid function in susceptible people.

Dietary supplements

The majority of vegetarians do not need supplements once their absorption mechanisms have had time to adjust to the new diet. During the first few months on the new diet there is a small risk of vitamin and mineral deficiency. A mild multivitamin and mineral supplement may be recommended during the transitional period.

Teenagers

Teenage vegetarians may be at risk of multiple deficiencies because of the extra nutrient requirements for growth, or because the diet is unbalanced. It is a wise precaution to recommend a mild multivitamin and mineral product, which includes 500 mg of calcium for all teenage vegetarians.

Vegans

Vegans are at risk of vitamin and mineral deficiency and a multivitamin and mineral supplement is advisable. It should contain vitamin B_{12} (unless fortified foods are consumed) and also iodine. If the product is for a child or a pregnant or breast-feeding woman, it should also contain vitamin D and calcium.

Care should be taken not to recommend products which contain amounts exceeding the RNI or RDA. Vitamin B_{12} is not absorbed orally in doses exceeding 3 µg, and excessive amounts of both vitamin D and iodine can be toxic. Many kelp preparations, for example, contain toxic concentrations of iodine.

Inactive ingredients

Dietary supplements recommended to vegetarians should be free from animal products. Capsules are normally made from gelatin but non-gelatin capsules are now available. Calcium may be derived from bones, and many vegetarians will also want to avoid lactose. Vitamin D may be derived from animal residues; vitamin D_{12} is acceptable, vitamin D_3 is not. Acceptable supplements are labelled as 'free from animal products' or 'suitable for vegetarians'.

In summary, a mild multivitamin and mineral supplement containing about the RNI or RDA for each nutrient should be recommended to the following groups of vegetarians:

- All vegans – adults and children
- All new vegetarians – for the first 6 months
- All teenage vegetarians

> **Dietary advice for vegetarians**
>
> (1) Convert to vegetarianism gradually – over several months – and take a multivitamin supplement during the transitional period
> (2) Replace meat and poultry with a mixture of pulses, nuts, soya products, e.g. textured vegetable protein (TVP), and eggs
> (3) Choose reduced-fat dairy products
> (4) Emphasise iron-rich plant foods, e.g. wholemeal bread, wholegrain cereals, pulses and green, leafy vegetables
> (5) Consume a source of vitamin C at each meal, e.g. citrus fruit or juice, tomatoes, green vegetables, salad, potatoes
> (6) Emphasise calcium-rich plant foods, e.g. green vegetables, nuts, pulses, sesame seeds and tofu. This advice is important for vegans; lacto-vegetarians obtain calcium from milk
> (7) Emphasise the importance of vitamin B_{12} fortified foods for vegans or use of a supplement
> (8) Emphasise the importance of products fortified with vitamin D, e.g. margarines and breakfast cereals (if acceptable)
> (9) Consider dietary supplements for vegans, especially those who are pregnant or breast feeding, children and teenage vegetarians

Further reading

National Dairy Council (1990) Nutrition and Vegetarianism. Fact File No 6. The National Dairy Council, London.

Useful addresses

The Vegan Society, 7 Battle Road, St Leonards-on-Sea, East Sussex TN37 7AA. Tel: 01424 427393.
The Vegetarian Society of the United Kingdom Ltd, Parkdale, Dunham Road, Altrincham, Cheshire WA14 4QG. Tel: 0161 925 2000.

Chapter 22
International Travel

Increasing numbers of people now leave the UK every year for holidays or business. Many suffer from ill health, and diarrhoea caused by contaminated food and water is all too common, affecting about 20–50% of all travellers. It is likely to cause distress and inconvenience and may even disrupt travel and business plans. For infants it is particularly serious, and may even be fatal if not treated promptly and effectively. Other food- and water-borne diseases which may be acquired by travellers to hot climates include cholera, typhoid, paratyphoid, hepatitis and various parasitic infections. Vaccination requirements should always be checked.

Food poisoning is not confined to hot climates: it also occurs in the UK (see Chapter 4). The general principles of food hygiene should always be followed but more detailed and specific advice should be given to travellers. Eating safely in a hot climate does not always mean eating foods which are considered to be healthy at home. Any nutritional benefit has to be weighed against microbiological risk. Fruit, for example, should be avoided unless it can be peeled. A can of cola and a plate of chips do not fit in with the current ideas of healthy heating, but at least they are likely to be microbiologically safe.

Specific hazards

Food

Careful selection and preparation of food are essential, but the appearance of food is no guide to the likelihood of contamination. Well cooked, piping hot food eaten immediately after preparation is generally safe, but cooked food held at room temperatures in tropical countries for several hours constitutes one of the greatest risks of food-borne disease, because bacteria can grow at phenomenal rates at these temperatures. Hotel buffets should be viewed with some suspicion.

Some foods pose more of a risk than others. These include various species of fish and shellfish which at certain times of the year contain poisonous biotoxins which are not even destroyed by thorough cooking. Shellfish in particular have long been associated with outbreaks of food poisoning and are best avoided.

Salads, raw vegetables and unpeeled fruit should not be eaten unless they can be washed with clean water. Unpasteurised milk, and yoghurt and ice cream made from it, should always be avoided.

Water and drinks

Water is a common source of contamination, and drinking tap water or any other untreated water from an unknown source is best avoided. This applies to water for food preparation and for cleaning teeth. Even bottled water and fruit drinks cannot automatically be assumed to be safe. Well known brand names of bottled waters and canned drinks should be chosen wherever possible, and opened in the presence of the consumer. Carbonated water is slightly safer than still water. Hot tea and coffee are usually safe, as are beer and wine, but alcoholic drinks can be dehydrating and should not be relied on for fluid intake in hot climates.

If tap water cannot be avoided it must be purified. This can be achieved by boiling, chemical sterilisation or filtration. Water must be boiled vigorously for five minutes; even at high altitude this is sufficient.

When boiling is not practicable, chemical sterilisation may be used. Either iodine or chlorine may be used. Both iodine-and chlorine-based disinfection preparations are available commercially, and manufacturer's instructions must be carefully followed. alternatively tincture of iodine (2%) may be used; five drops should be added to 1 litre of water. Chemically treated water should be left to stand for half an hour and must be clear before use.

Filtration can also be used when boiling is not practicable. Various filters and filtration bags (e.g. Millbank Bags, Johnson Progress Ltd) are available for this purpose. Needless to say, the manufacturer's instructions should always be followed closely. Filtered water should never be given to babies and young children without boiling or disinfection. Water purifiers (e.g. Portapure, Porta Products Ltd) which purify large volumes of water at once are also available. Advice for travellers is summarised below:

Food and drink advice for travellers.

(1) Drink bottled water purchased in sealed containers; carbonated water is safer than still

(2) Avoid tap water unless it is boiled or sterilised

(3) Avoid ice in drinks

(4) Hot tea, coffee, canned fizzy drinks, cartons of fruit juice, and beer and wine are generally safe

(5) Choose food that is freshly cooked and piping hot; avoid food which has obviously been kept warm

(6) Avoid salads, and raw vegetables and fruit unless they can be peeled by the consumer

(7) Avoid unpasteurised milk

(8) Avoid ice cream and ices

(9) Avoid shellfish

(10) Take a multivitamin supplement if travelling to a country (for a period of longer than a month) where the diet is substantially different from the habitual diet

Chapter 23
Cultural Diversity

Britain contains a rich diversity of people. In 1991 the total ethnic minority population was just over 3 million, representing 5.5% of the total population. About half of these people were born in Britain.

The largest minority ethnic groups are the Asians and Afro-Caribbeans. Substantial immigration from the West Indies started in the 1950s in response to post-war labour shortages in Britain. This was followed in the 1960s by groups of people from India, Pakistan (formerly West Pakistan) and Bangladesh (formerly East Pakistan), and in the 1970s by Indians from East Africa.

Most live in Greater London and the Metropolitan counties of England (see Table 23.1) where employment opportunities were greatest at the time of arrival. In addition there are large communities in Blackburn, Leicester, Luton, Nottingham and Slough.

Table 23.1 Percentage population of ethnic minorities in specific areas of Great Britain (1991 Census).

Ethnic group	Great Britain	Greater London	Greater Manchester	West Yorkshire	West Midlands Metropolitan Council	East Midlands
Indian	1.5	5.2	1.2	1.7	5.5	2.5
Bangladeshi	0.3	1.3	0.5	0.3	0.7	0.1
Pakistani	0.9	1.3	2.0	4.0	3.5	0.4
Afro-Caribbean	0.9	4.4	0.7	0.7	2.8	0.6
Chinese	0.3	0.8	0.3	0.2	0.2	0.2
African	0.4	2.4	0.2	0.1	0.2	0.1
Total ethnic minorities[1]	5.5	20.2	5.9	8.2	14.6	4.8

[1] Totals are different from the sum of groups shown because some ethnic groups are not included.

Members of cultural minorities experience a number of social disadvantages (e.g. high unemployment) compared with other groups. These difficulties may be compounded by relative unfamiliarity with British society and, especially among Asian groups, by differences in language and culture. Disruptions associated with migration are likely to influence health and may impose imbalances in the diet. Pharmacists should be aware of these difficulties; discrimination can often be unintentional.

Asians

In Britain the term Asian is used to represent people from India, Pakistan and Bangladesh. Most Indians living in Britain have come from Gujarat and the Punjab, although most of the Gujaratis came to Britain after a period in East Africa. India covers an enormous geographical area, and among Asians there is a great variety of language, religion, culture and dietary practice. The family remains a strong institution.

Dietary practices are influenced by both religion and culture (see Table 23.2). Fasting is a requirement of some religions. There is also a considerable emphasis on social events which involve gathering together and eating. Festivals occur frequently, and, as in many celebrations, these often involve rich and refined foods which are high in fat and sugar.

Gujaratis

Religion and language

Most Gujaratis are Hindus. A small number belong to the Jain sect which resembles Buddhism. A few are Muslims, Christians or Buddhists. Gujarati and Hindi are the main languages.

Naming system

Most Gujaratis have a first name, a middle name and a family or sub-caste name. Common family names include Patel and Shah. The traditional form of address is by first and middle name only, but title and family name (e.g. Mr Patel) are acceptable in the UK.

Diet

The staple diet is usually chapatti which is an unleavened bread. Ghee (clarified butter) is the most common form of fat used but vegetable oil is acceptable in some recipes. Dairy products and pulses are important foods in the diet.

What is excluded from the diet depends to some extent on the strictness of adherence to the religion which, as has already been pointed out, is normally Hindu. The practice of non-violence against living things means that many Hindus are vegetarian. Strict Hindus exclude eggs, and some may avoid cheese if it is made from animal rennet. Other Hindus eat some meat but all avoid meat from the cow, which is considered to be sacred. Alcohol is officially frowned on.

Table 23.2 General dietary patterns of the main Asian groups in Britain.

Country of origin	Staple cereal	Meat	Fish	Pulses	Fats	Dairy products	Eggs	Fruit and vegetables
India								
Gujarat								
Hindus	Chapattis or rice	No beef; usually vegetarian	Little	Very important	Ghee or oil	Important	Not eaten by strict vegetarians	Important
Muslims	Chapattis or rice	No pork; halal meat only	Little	Important	Ghee or oil	Important	Some	Important
Punjab[1]								
Sikhs	Chapattis	No beef; some vegetarian	None	Very important	Ghee	Very important	Very few	Important
Hindus	Chapattis	No beef; usually vegetarian	None	Very important	Ghee	Very important	Not eaten by strict vegetarians	Important
Bangladesh								
Muslims	Rice	No pork; halal meat only	Important	Important	Oil or some ghee	Few	Few	Important
Pakistan								
Muslims	Chapattis	No pork; halal meat only	Little	Important	Ghee or oil	Important	Some	Important

[1] Some Punjabis in Britain are from Pakistan and are Muslims.
Adapted from Health Education Authority (1991).

Punjabis

Religion and language

Most Punjabis coming from India are Sikhs but a few are Hindus. Some Punjabis are from the Pakistani state of Punjab and are Muslims. All of them speak Punjabi.

Naming system

Sikhs generally have a first name followed by a religious name which in men is Singh and in women Kaur. In addition they sometimes use a family name. The traditional form of address is the first name and the religious name together, although 'Mr Singh' is acceptable to some.

Diet

Chapattis are the staple food in the Punjab, and considerable importance is placed on pulses and dairy products. The dietary customs of Sikhs overlap with those of Hindus and Muslims. In practice they are largely vegetarian, and, although some eat meat, few eat beef. Alcohol is forbidden, but this regulation is sometimes ignored.

Bangladeshis and Pakistanis

Religion and language

Almost all Bangladeshis and Pakistanis are Muslims. Those from Bangladesh speak Bengali; those from Pakistan speak Urdu and Punjabi.

Naming system

The naming system is quite complicated, and men and women have different systems. Men have a religious name (i.e. Muslim title) which may be the first name listed and a personal name. They may also have a family name, but these are not commonly used. Religious names include Abdul, Allah, Muhammad, Syed and Ullah. The most acceptable form of address is the Muslim title followed by the personal name.

Women usually have two names including a personal name followed by a female title such as Bibi, Begum or Khattoon. The title should not be used in isolation; it is meaningless to say 'Mrs Bibi'.

Diet

The staple cereals in Bangladesh and Pakistan are rice and chapattis respectively. Fish is popular in Bangladesh but less so in Pakistan.

Muslims may eat meat but it must be 'halal', i.e. slaughtered according to the prescribed method and the blood drained. Pig meat is excluded. All alcoholic drinks, and dishes including alcohol, are prohibited.

Fasting

Muslims are required to fast during the month of Ramadan which is the ninth month of the Muslim calendar. The date varies slightly each year. The fast lasts from sunrise to sunset each day and involves abstinence from all food and drink. People exempted from the fast include children who have not reached puberty, the elderly, women who are menstruating, pregnant or breast feeding and those who are ill or on a journey. The expectation is that these people will make up the fast whenever possible.

Drug compliance may be a problem during Ramadan and the whole day's dose of medicine may be taken with the evening meal. In some cases, pharmacists may be able to recommend alternative medication to the GP. For example, a single night-time dose of a modified-release formulation may suffice. Patients can then receive satisfactory treatment whilst abiding by their religious convictions. There is generally no restriction on the use of inhalers, injections, suppositories or skin preparations.

Traditional Asian medicine

Pharmacists should be aware that Asian patients may be using alternative medicines as well as those prescribed. Traditional healers are popular, not only because their treatments are believed to be effective, but also because they speak the same language as the patient and understand their culture.

Ayurvedic medicine

The philosophy behind the traditional Ayurvedic system of medicine is that disease is brought about by an imbalance in what are described as the 'humours' of the body. These are fire, which is characterised as hot, air, which is dry and water, which is cold. Treatment of disease aims to restore the balance of these characteristics. Food, medicine and illness are classified according to the presence or absence of these components. Meat, fish, nuts, spices and some pulses are considered 'hot' while fruits, vegetables and dairy products are 'cold'. If the disease is considered to be a 'hot' condition, 'cold' foods will be prescribed and vice versa. This practice is likely to influence nutrition.

Ayurvedic remedies are not licensed medicines and are freely available in some Indian supermarkets. Some contain toxic levels of heavy metals such as arsenic, cadmium, lead and mercury, which may cause unpleasant side-effects and long-term damage. Herbs are also used. Karela, for example, lowers blood glucose and may be used in diabetes mellitus; it may interfere with the action of oral hypoglycaemics. The Asian community in the UK should be made aware of the risks associated with some traditional remedies.

Paan

Chewing paan is still widely practised particularly by older members of the Asian community. Paan contains betel nut and other ingredients wrapped up in a betel leaf, and is used as a digestive aid and breath freshener. It may cause mouth inflammation, dental decay and possibly cancer, and may also interact with prescribed medicines.

Nutritional problems

The traditional Asian diet of chapattis and rice with vegetables and, for non-vegetarians, small amounts of meat or fish is basically the type of diet which is now recommended for all British people. It is not unhealthy; where problems do occur they are more likely to be the result of adopting Western eating habits.

The higher incidence of coronary heart disease and non-insulin dependent diabetes mellitus in the Asian community is a cause for concern. These findings are not adequately explained by ethnic differences in conventional risk factors, such as smoking, hypertension and raised serum cholesterol levels. They may be related to diet but could also be a result of genetic factors and, in the present older generation, by the stress of migration and unfamiliarity with British society.

Vitamin D deficiency

Vitamin D deficiency leads to rickets in children and osteomalacia in adults, both of which are found in the Asian community in Britain, although the incidence, at least of rickets, appears to be falling. Most vitamin D is obtained by the action of sunlight on the skin, but the cultural practice of covering the skin and staying indoors which is observed by some Asian women is likely to limit the amount of vitamin D synthesised in the skin.

Dietary vitamin D is obtained mainly from animal foods, and many Asians are vegetarians. Margarine which is fortified by law with the vitamin is not widely used in the Asian community. Chapattis are often blamed because of their high phytate content, which may interfere with vitamin D metabolism.

Iron deficiency

Anaemia does occur in Asians in both adults and children but the reasons for it are not very clear. The fact that many are vegetarians may increase the risk.

The provision of an adequate diet for Asian infants in Great Britain can be a problem, due to the difficulty of obtaining weaning foods prepared according to religious laws and because of uncertainty as to whether commercial food has been handled appropriately or contains forbidden ingredients. The use of commercial baby foods therefore tends to be limited to sweets and fruits. These are low in iron.

There may be an over-reliance on milk, particularly cow's milk which is low in iron. If the mother is not breast feeding, a follow-on formula (see Chapter 16) should be recommended over the age of 6 months. Most rusks and baby cereals are also fortified with iron.

Dietary advice

Food habits are changing in the Asian community and dietary advice must take into account the extent to which the individual has adopted Western eating patterns. This depends on factors such as ability to communicate, employment of the mother outside the home, peer group pressure at school, and exposure to the media, all of which relate to the level of social interaction with the wider community.

Increasing length of stay in Britain may be associated with greater dietary change, but sometimes the reverse is true. During the 1960s the availability of traditional foods was minimal, and the cost, especially of what were then unusual fruits and vegetables in Britain, was prohibitive. Traditional foods are now more widely available.

Breakfast is the meal where most marked changes have occurred. Convenience is a prime consideration at breakfast and it is also the meal of least symbolic significance. Western breakfast of toast and cereals is therefore widely adopted. Changes to midday meal patterns depend on the extent to which family members are out at work or school. A traditional meal is more likely to be eaten in the evening since this is when the family often eat together.

Dietary advice needs to be based on a thorough knowledge of the foods eaten, of dietary practices and of the language; a generalist approach must be avoided. This will be beyond the skills of many pharmacists, but the following advice may be considered:

- Using brown chapatti flour
- Emphasising the importance of pulses
- Reducing the amount of ghee used in cooking or replacing with vegetable oil in appropriate recipes
- Reducing the intake of sweet pickles
- Reducing the intake of sweets and the use of gur (unrefined sugar) in cooking

Any advice given must be culturally acceptable. Advising Asians to cut out ghee is likely to fall on deaf ears; it is an important cooking ingredient and many traditional foods taste unpleasant without it. But the amount can be reduced and vegetable oil can be used in some recipes. Similarly, sweets are an important part of Asian festivals and family gatherings, and there is no point in advising that they be excluded. Recipes can often be adapted and amounts of sugar reduced. Some typical Asian foods are shown in Table 23.3.

Table 23.3   Some Asian foods.

Breads		*Savoury snacks (fried)*	
Bhakari	Paratha	Bhajia	Pakora
Chapatti	Poppadom	Chevda	Samosa
Naan	Puri	Ganthia	

Sweet snacks	
Burfi	Ladoos
Gulab Jamen	Ras Gulas
Jellabi	Shira
Kheer	Shrikand

Pulses and dhals (with alternative names)
(Dhal = lentil-based dish)

Bengal gram; channa dhal; chickpea
Masur dhal; red lentil
Green gram; moong (pronounced 'muck') dhal; mung bean
Red gram; toor dhal; pigeon pea
Matar dhal; split pea
Black gram; urad dhal

The richness of the culinary heritage of the Asian community means that with some adjustment the diet can be very healthy. Traditional dietary patterns should be encouraged and, if desired, combined with Western foods based on the healthy eating guidelines in Chapter 3.

Afro-Caribbeans

Origins and culture

Afro-Caribbeans are people of African origin who came to Britain from the Caribbean islands. English is universally spoken and many are Christians, which means that their diets are free from religious restrictions.

An increasing number of young Afro-Caribbeans are Rastafarians, some of whom are vegetarian and others vegans. Foods containing additives and preservatives are likely to be avoided by Rastafarians.

Diet

The diet is based on staple cereals such as wheat, rice and maize; roots and tubers such as yams, cassava and sweet potatoes; plantain (green bananas); and breadfruit. Meats such as chicken and goat are popular, as is salt pork and salt fish; indeed salt fish with ackee (a vegetable) is a national favourite.

Fried foods are enjoyed and butter is often added to vegetables after cooking. Some traditional ingredients are high in fat, e.g. creamed coconut. Ackee and avocado are often thought to be low in fat because they are fruits, but one medium avocado contains about 30 g of fat and a portion of ackee about 15 g of fat.

Nutritional problems

Afro-Caribbeans suffer from iron deficiency but to a lesser extent than Asians. The Afro-Caribbean community shows a high incidence of stroke and hypertension; maintaining ideal body weight and reducing salt intake may help in preventing these disorders.

Dietary advice

In addition to the guidelines in Chapter 3, the following advice should be considered:

- Encouraging the consumption of starchy fruit and vegetables as part of the main meal, e.g. yams, cassava, sweet potato, plantain, breadfruit, but not frying them
- Avoiding or reducing the amount of creamed coconut in cooking, or replacing with yoghurt
- Limiting the consumption of avocado and ackee
- Soaking salt fish and salt meat in water for 1–2 hours to remove excess salt
- Saving Caribbean delicacies (e.g. sweet potato pie) for special occasions.

Jewish people

Judaism is an ancient religion and Jewish religious practices are laid down in the Torah (the first five books of the Bible) and the Talmud.

Dietary regulations

The Jewish dietary regulations are observed to varying degrees by all practising Jews; they do not pose any particular risks to health.

Pork and its derivatives are forbidden, as are shellfish. Meat from animals with a cloven hoof and which chew the cud are allowed, e.g. cows, sheep, goat. Fish with fins and scales are permitted. Birds of prey are forbidden, but chicken, turkey, pheasant, pigeon, goose and partridge are allowed.

Meat and dairy products must not be served or cooked together, and must not be eaten within several hours of each other. Separate plates and utensils must be used for them. All animals and birds must be slaughtered by the prescribed Jewish method to render them kosher (permitted). The salt content of kosher meat if often higher than that of non-kosher meat. If a low-salt diet is prescribed, the meat can be soaked to remove excess salt.

Medicines

Orthodox Jews avoid non-kosher medicines unless there are not alternatives; some additives are also unacceptable to Jewish people. Information about kosher medicines is available from Rabbi A. Adler (consultant pharmacist to the London and Manchester Beth Din), 172 Whitehall Road, Gateshead, Tyne and Wear NE8 1TP.

There are several Jewish festivals, and some involve fasting, e.g. Yom Kippur (Day of Atonement). Orthodox patients may require alternatives to oral medication, such as suppositories or injections.

Further reading

Health and Ethnicity Programme (1991) *The Ethnic Health Factfile. A guide for health professionals who care for people from ethnic backgrounds.* North West/ North East Thames Region Health Authority, London.

Health Education Authority (1991) *Nutrition in Minority Ethnic Groups, Asians and Afro-Caribbeans in the United Kingdom.* The Health Education Authority, London.

Healy, M.A. & Aslam M. (1989) *The Asian Community – Medicines and Traditions.* Silver Link Publishing, Peterborough.

Tan, S.P., Wenlock, R.W. & Buss, D.H. (1985) Immigrant foods. 2nd supplement to *McCance and Widdowson's The Composition of Foods.* HMSO, London.

Chapter 24
Low Income

All healthy adults should be encouraged to eat a healthy diet (see Chapter 3), but sensitivity is required towards those on low incomes because they will find some of the guidelines (e.g. increasing fruit intake) extremely difficult to follow. Most health professionals take for granted an ability to choose a healthy diet if desired, but this is not so for those on low incomes.

People on low incomes constitute a diverse group with differing needs and constraints. They include single-parent families, the long-term unemployed, the homeless, students, those in bed and breakfast and other temporary accommodation, some elderly people and some members of ethnic groups.

Health

Disadvantaged groups suffer more ill health than the better off. Problems such as low birthweight, poor dental health, obesity and cardiovascular disorders are all more common in these groups. Poor diet is a contributory factor, but poor housing, lack of morale and constant financial worry are equally important.

Diet

Cost of healthy eating

It is often argued that a healthy diet need be no more expensive than an unhealthy one, but whether it is within the reach of people who are on social security benefits is another matter. While the average UK family spends 12.4% of income on food eaten at home, the poorest may spend nearly 50%. The cost of eating healthily would increase this proportion still further. And when money is short, food is usually the first item to be cut down.

Poor people do not have any room for manoeuvre. The proportion of income devoted to fixed costs, such as housing and fuel, means that the only way that poor people can increase their spending is to fall into debt. In 1991 this was a problem affecting 2.6 million households.

What do poor people eat?

Low income households tend to satisfy their appetites on cheap, energy-dense foods which are high in fat and sugar and low in non-starch polysaccharides. In terms of calories, poor people get very good value for money but at the cost of a healthy diet. To obtain 100 calories from two custard creams costs 3 pence, but 35 pence to obtain the same number of calories from oranges.

Poor people eat less cheese and lean meat than the better off, but one of the most striking differences in the diet of the poor is the low intake of fruit and fresh vegetables; they simply cannot afford them. The cost of providing two or three pieces of fruit per day for each person in a family of six on income support is impossible.

The diets of poor people are therefore likely not only to be high in fat and sugar but low in fibre, folic acid and the anti-oxidant nutrients (e.g. beta-carotene and vitamin C). This is important, because evidence suggests that lack of anti-oxidant nutrients is associated with disease such as cancer and cardiovascular disease.

Food choice

Factors other than health govern everybody's choice of food (see Chapter 1), but this is even more so for those on low incomes. Income is certainly a major factor, but availability of food, cooking facilities, ease of preparation and family acceptability are interlinked and equally important.

Food purchase

Food shopping has changed out of all recognition in recent years, and the once weekly or even once monthly shop at a supermarket has become the norm for most people. However, for many poor people living on housing estates in the inner cities, travelling to supermarkets is not practicable. Taking several young children on a bus is very stressful, and although the cost per item may be less the tendency is often to spend far more. Those living in temporary accommodation do not have storage facilities for large amounts of food and cannot take advantage of bulk buying. If cooking facilities are poor or non-existent, they may use take-aways or local cafés.

Although many poor people do shop weekly or fortnightly – the day they obtain their income support – this tends to be at the nearest and cheapest local store. Choice, particularly of healthy alternatives such as low fat spreads, may be limited in these shops.

Food preparation

Cooking facilities may be a limiting factor for people on poor incomes. In bed and breakfast accommodation there are likely to be queues for the kitchen, and cooking from raw ingredients is simply not practicable. Cooking fish may well be unpopular in cramped conditions because of the lingering smell. Soaking and cooking pulses is time consuming and messy; canned pulses are expensive. Chips are quicker to cook than boiled potatoes and crisps need no cooking at all.

Lack of confidence and fear of waste prevent many mothers from cooking with basic ingredients. Buying herbs and flour for a recipe which is only tried once is expensive. If the family refuses to eat the meal, there is no money for another one, so it is far easier to buy sausages and burgers which the children will definitely eat.

Attitudes

Many poor people find their diet boring and repetitive. It is not that they want to eat like this. A few may lack organisational and budgeting skills, but contrary to popular belief many poor people know what is meant by a healthy diet. Most would like to buy more fruit, salad, cheese and lean meat, but lack of money, low morale and the psychological and social factors already discussed militate against this. Short-term worries, such as paying the bills, tend to overwhelm any longer term concerns about health.

Advice

Pharmacists will have very few opportunities to give dietary advice to people on low incomes. One thing they can do is to make sure that any low income households with which they have contact are in receipt of all the benefits to which they are entitled. Lack of money rather than information is the main barrier to improving eating habits in poor people. The benefits system changes regularly, and pharmacists, particularly those practising in areas of deprivation, should keep up to date.

Healthy eating concepts are often inappropriate but it is worth encouraging:

- Budgeting for and purchasing the most important food items first, e.g. bread, potatoes, cereals, milk
- Sharing shopping trips with friends and neighbours to reduce the sense of isolation and make better use of transport facilities
- Encouraging local co-operatives for food shopping; some health centres have set up discount food stores selling healthy food items
- Fostering local initiatives to encourage group discussion of healthy eating and trying out new recipes to increase confidence and cooking skills
- Encouraging the consumption of pizzas and jacket potatoes as take-aways rather than pies and chips.

Further reading

Health Education Authority (1989) *Diet, Nutrition and 'Healthy Eating' in Low Income Groups.* Health Education Authority. London.

National Consumer Council (1992) *Your Food: Whose Choice?* HMSO, London.

Useful addresses

Child Poverty Action Group, 4th Floor, 1–5 Bath Street, London EC1V 9PY. Tel: 0207 253 3406.

Section 6
Drugs and Nutrition

Chapter 25
Dietary Supplements

The fact that vitamins and minerals are important in the maintenance of good health is undeniable; and at least one in four adults now takes some form of food supplement. While vitamin deficiency is a risk in some groups of the population, these tend not to be the people who buy supplements. Many supplements are bought in the absence of any clear signs of deficiency.

Expectations of benefits from supplements may be unrealistic. Individuals with serious illness are quite naturally attracted by the hope of freedom from disease, and one of the dangers of supplements is that they may be used in the place of conventional medical care. Other reasons for purchase include lack of energy, susceptibility to colds, hair loss and dry skin.

Supplements are not necessarily as innocuous as is often believed; some can be as toxic as drugs in overdose. However, the majority of people do not treat them as a form of medication and are unaware of the potential harm of inappropriate administration. Advice should always be given abut dosage.

Some supplements interact with drugs and could reduce beneficial therapeutic effects (see Chapter 26). Others should be used with caution or avoided in certain situations (e.g. excessive vitamin A in pregnancy). When asking patients questions about their medicines, or responding to symptoms, pharmacists should always specifically ask if dietary supplements are being taken.

Pharmacists have more contact with people buying dietary supplements than any other health professionals, and have a responsibility to educate the public in their safe and rational use.

What are dietary supplements?

Dietary supplements are products which contain nutrients or other ingredients which consumers believe to have particularly beneficial effects on their health. They are known as 'diet integrators' in EU law.

There are several categories of dietary supplements including:

- Vitamins and minerals
- Health supplements, e.g. fish liver oils
- Slimming products (see Chapter 19)

- Food supplements, e.g. Build-Up and Complan (see Chapter 28)
- Fortified foods, e.g. bread, margarine, breakfast cereals.

This chapter discusses vitamins and minerals and health supplements. It does not cover herbal and homoeopathic supplements; these are beyond the scope of this book.

Legal status

The majority of dietary supplements are not licensed medicines and they do not have product licences; they are classified as foods. Dietary supplements are therefore exempt from the controls of the Medicines Act.

This means that they are not subject to the same sale and supply restrictions as licensed medicines. Licensed medicines containing vitamins A and D, cyanocobalamin and folic acid are categorised as prescription only (POM), pharmacy only (P) or general sales list (GSL) depending on the maximum daily dose recommended on the product label, as shown in Table 25.1.

Table 25.1 Limitations on the sale or supply of licensed medicines containing certain vitamins.

Vitamins	Legal status
Vitamin A	Up to 2250 µg (7500 IU) GSL Over 2250 µg (7500 IU) POM
Vitamin D	Up to 10 µg (400 IU) GSL Over 10 µg (400 IU) P
Cyanocobalamin	Up to 10 µg GSL Over 10 µg P
Folic acid	Up to 200 µg GSL 200–500 µg P Over 500 µg POM

A dietary supplement is not subject to any of these sale and supply restrictions even if it contains those vitamins listed in Table 25.1 in excess of the daily dose limitations. It is possible, say, to buy dietary supplements containing 7.5 mg (25 000 IU) of vitamin A or 1000 µg of folic acid. Dietary supplements may contain more, less, or exactly the same amount of an active ingredient as a prescription only medicine.

Labelling

Dietary supplements are subject to different labelling regulations from those that relate to licensed medicines. Because they are classified as foods, dietary supplements must be labelled according to the Food Labelling Regulations, whereas medicines must be labelled according to the regulations of the Medicines Act.

Labels on supplements must include a full list of ingredients, including additives and excipients. Some are labelled as being 'free from animal products' or 'suitable for vegetarians'. This can be a useful feature particularly for individuals who are trying to avoid certain substances, e.g. lactose.

Claims

Unlike licensed medicines, dietary supplements may not be promoted for medicinal use. In other words, no claim – either direct or implied – may be made that a dietary supplement is 'capable of preventing, treating or curing human disease'. Thus, the labelling of a dietary supplement with the claim that 'this product can be used to prevent heart disease' or that 'this product reduces the risk of thrombosis' is an offence.

On the face of it, this prohibition ought to protect the public from misleading claims. Yet it is well known that many people have extraordinary expectations of dietary supplements. How does this happen?

Part of the answer to this lies in the fact that it is often difficult in law to decide whether a dietary supplement is claiming a medicinal use or not. Claims such as 'this product may help to reduce the risk of hypertension' may be quite naturally interpreted by the public to mean that such a product will prevent or cure high blood pressure. A product labelled 'may lower cholesterol' could be taken to mean that the product will give definite protection against heart attacks. One of the greatest dangers of such misleading claims is that they may encourage people to abandon prescribed medication or avoid it in the first place. Pharmacists should, when the opportunity arises, warn people about the risks of relying on such claims.

Claims such as 'this product can help to maintain a healthy heart' or 'several people report improved energy levels with this product' are interpreted in law as health claims and are permissible for dietary supplements. The important distinction between a medicinal claim and a health claim is that a health claim makes no mention of disease treatment or prevention. Health claims can however refer to body organs or body systems.

While it is possible to restrict claims made in the labelling and advertising of a dietary supplement, no such restrictions apply to authors of books and magazine articles and these are often sold alongside supplements. Authors are perfectly free to express their own opinions and it is books and articles which are the source of many people's mistaken ideas.

Most members of the public are not in a position to distinguish between direct medicinal claims, implied medicinal claims, health claims and the opinions of authors. Pharmacists should be aware of this confusion and be prepared to correct any misconceptions. However, the food industry, the regulatory bodies and consumer groups are working together in the UK on a claims initiative. This, and new directives from the European Union, should help to clarify this situation in the future.

Formulation

Dietary supplements are available in the form of tablets, capsules, liquids and powders. Solid dose preparations are available in chewable, effervescent and slow-release forms. Some contain nutrients in a 'chelated' form which is thought to improve absorption. However, there is little to choose between any of these formulations. Natural products are no more efficacious than synthetic ones; whether synthetically or naturally derived all nutrients are absorbed according to the same mechanisms. Vitamin E is one exception where the natural form is more bioavailable than the synthetic form.

Quality control over food supplements is currently far less exacting than it is over medicines. Medicines have to be tested for consistent dosage levels, disintegration standards and bioavailability. There is some evidence that the concentration of vitamins and minerals in dietary supplements varies considerably from that stated on the label. More rigorous standards for purity may be developed in the future.

Vitamins and minerals

Vitamins and minerals are essential substances which are required in daily amounts ranging from micrograms to milligrams (see Appendix 1). Vitamins are either fat-soluble (A, D, E and K) or water-soluble (B group and C).

Most vitamins must be acquired from the diet because they cannot be synthesised by the body. A few vitamins can be synthesised in the body, and this provides amounts in addition to the diet. Vitamin D is synthesised in the skin in considerable amounts after exposure to sunlight. Vitamin K and biotin are synthesised by the intestinal flora. The B vitamin niacin is formed *in vivo* from the amino acid tryptophan, and vitamin A is formed from its precursor beta-carotene.

In general, vitamins and minerals function as part of enzyme systems and in the structure of tissues such as bone and blood. They may also play specific roles in the prevention of disease beyond the classic deficiency disorders such as scurvy. Examples include folic acid in the prevention of neural tube defects and the anti-oxidant nutrients, beta-carotene, selenium and vitamins C and E, in the prevention of coronary heart disease and cancer. The role of the anti-oxidant nutrients is under active investigation and it is still too early to make firm recommendations as to the value of supplements.

Overt vitamin and mineral deficiencies are relatively rare in the UK, but there is a risk of subclinical deficiency in some groups of the population (e.g. the elderly). When deficiencies do occur they are seldom isolated. This is because a diet poor in one nutrient is usually poor in several others.

The clinical development of vitamin deficiencies is usually gradual, and early symptoms are general and unspecific. Tiredness, hair loss and general malaise, typically attributed to vitamin deficiency, can be observed in several disorders and could easily be due to other causes such as bereavement or stress. The possibility of more serious disease should not be overlooked; hair loss, for example, could be indicative of a thyroid disorder. Such symptoms should not be taken to mean that a specific nutrient is missing from the diet. A number of clinical tests are required to confirm deficiency.

Details of dietary sources, functions and deficiency symptoms of vitamins and minerals can be found in Appendix 2.

Vitamin and mineral preparations are used extensively in the practice of medicine and are valuable when used properly. It is important that a clear distinction is made between their use as therapeutic agents and their use as dietary supplements.

Therapeutic agents

Vitamins and minerals can be prescribed on the NHS for the prevention and treatment of specific deficiency in certain situations including:

- Malabsorption conditions, such as Crohn's disease, ulcerative colitis and cystic fibrosis (see Chapter 8), coeliac disease (see Chapter 9)
- Anaemia (see Chapter 10)
- Renal disease (see Chapter 11)
- Liver disease (see Chapter 12)
- Rickets and osteomalacia (see Chapter 13)
- The long-term administration of some drugs, e.g. anticonvulsants (see Chapter 26)
- Wernicke's encephalopathy and Korsakoff's psychosis, which are often seen in chronic alcoholics and are caused by vitamin B deficiency.

In all these situations vitamins and minerals should be prescribed by the GP.

Vitamins are also used as pharmacological agents for certain non-nutritional disease states. If dosage of a vitamin is increased beyond the physiological range, no further physiological action is expected, but pharmacological actions may occur.

Pharmacological doses of vitamin A exert an anti-proliferative effect on the skin, and derivatives of vitamin A (retinoids) have been developed which are used to treat some skin conditions (see Chapter 14). In doses of 150 times the Reference Nutrient Intake (RNI) nicotinic acid is used for the treatment of hyperlipidaemias.

Dietary supplements

There are three categories of vitamin and mineral supplements (see Table 25.2). The majority of people in the UK who eat a balanced diet do not need to take vitamin and mineral supplements. In response to requests for dietary supplements, pharmacists should always ask questions about the diet and give advice based on current healthy eating guidelines (see Chapter 3). Dietary supplements do not turn an unhealthy diet into a healthy one.

Table 25.2   Types of vitamin and mineral supplements.

(1)   Multivitamins and multiminerals. These usually contain around 100% of the Recommended Daily Amount (RDA) for each vitamin. If the product contains minerals, these are present in varying amounts
(2)   Combinations of particular vitamins and minerals marketed for specific groups of people such as schoolchildren, slimmers, menopausal women and athletes
(3)   Single vitamins or single minerals often containing very large amounts. When levels of vitamins and minerals exceed 10 times the RDA, they are usually known as 'megadoses'

All supplements are labelled in terms of the European Recommended Daily Amount (RDA) which is quantitatively similar to the Reference Nutrient Intake (RNI)

There are some groups of the population who are at risk of deficiency and might benefit from vitamin and mineral supplements. These include:

- Pregnant and breast feeding women (see Chapter 15)
- Infants (see Chapter 16)
- Children and young people (see Chapter 17)
- The elderly (see Chapter 18)
- Slimmers (see Chapter 19)
- Athletes (see Chapter 20)
- Vegetarians, particularly vegans (see Chapter 21)
- Long-term travellers (for periods longer than a month) to countries where the diet is substantially different from the habitual diet (see Chapter 22)
- Members of the Asian community, particularly during pregnancy, lactation, infancy and childhood (see Chapter 23)
- People on low incomes (see Chapter 24)

The best choice of dietary supplement for any of these groups of people is one which contains a wide variety of vitamins and minerals and which does not contain more than the Reference Nutrient Intake (RNI) of each nutrient.

Specific claims for vitamins and minerals

Megadoses of vitamins and minerals have been advocated in the treatment and prevention of a number of disorders where no proven deficiency exists. Pharmacists need some knowledge of these claims because they may be asked to explain them.

Vitamin A

Vitamin A is involved in the growth and differentiation of epithelial tissue, and it is a reasonable assumption that it might prevent and treat various skin disorders. However, results from trials of vitamin A in acne and other skin conditions have not provided enough evidence to justify its administration for these purposes. The use of pharmacological doses of vitamin A derivatives (retinoids) in skin conditions should not be confused with the use of vitamin A as a supplement.

Low intakes of both vitamin A and beta-carotene have been associated with an increased risk of cancer at various sites including the stomach, breast and respiratory tract. There appears to be an inverse relationship between serum vitamin A levels and various cancers, but associations do not prove causation, and there is not enough evidence at the moment to suggest that large doses of either vitamin A or beta-carotene prevent cancer. Indeed, some studies have shown a positive association between beta-carotene supplementation and the incidence of lung cancer.

Vitamin B$_6$

Megadoses of vitamin B$_6$ have been recommended for a variety of disorders including carpal tunnel syndrome, pregnancy sickness and asthma. Further research is necessary to confirm these effects. Again, the results are controversial, but pyridoxine appears to help some women with premenstrual syndrome.

Niacin

The term niacin covers both nicotinamide and nicotinic acid. Nicotinic acid is licensed in the UK as a lipid-lowering drug, but it should not be recommended as a dietary supplement for this purpose. Niacin was the first vitamin to be used by orthomolecular psychiatrists in the treatment of schizophrenia but evidence for such a beneficial effect has not been confirmed in controlled studies.

Folic acid

Low levels of folic acid are associated with neural tube defects, e.g. spina bifida in infants. All women who are pregnant or intend to become so should take a folic acid supplement (see Chapter 15). Increasingly, low folate status is also linked with increased risk of cardiovascular disease. Although the evidence is not yet conclusive, it is likely that a daily supplemental intake of 200–400 µg of folic acid could be beneficial. Evidence is also emerging that folic acid is beneficial in reducing the risk of colon cancer, and possibly also Alzheimer's disease, although clinical trials are needed.

Vitamin C

A beneficial effect of megadoses of vitamin C has been claimed for an extraordinary number of conditions including the common cold, wounds and cancer. Whilst vitamin C appears to reduce the severity of cold symptoms, this does not justify 'megadose' intakes.

Vitamin D

Few claims have been made for the benefits of large doses of vitamin D except in the treatment of deficiency. Vitamin D plays an essential role in the regulation of plasma calcium and in bone mineralisation and may be useful in the prevention and treatment of osteoporosis (see Chapter 13).

Vitamin E

The primary role of vitamin E is as an anti-oxidant helping to protect the tissues from free radical damage. Free radicals may be important in the development of cancer, and since vitamin E acts as a free radical scavenger it has been advocated in cancer prevention. Some studies show that the relative risk of developing cancer is higher in individuals with poor vitamin E status. At the present time, however, there is not enough evidence to recommend large doses of vitamin E for the prevention of cancer.

Large doses of vitamin E have also been advocated in cardiovascular disease There is some evidence that vitamin E has an effect in angina or in reducing serum cholesterol levels, and it may have a role in the prevention of thrombosis and also in intermittent claudication.

Calcium

The use of calcium supplements in the prevention and treatment of osteoporosis is described in Chapter 13. Calcium has also been claimed to lower blood pressure, but it should not be taken for this purpose without medical referral. If a patient is taking antihypertensive drugs, control of blood pressure could be prejudiced by the use of a calcium supplement.

Magnesium

Magnesium supplements have been promoted for a number of conditions including premenstrual syndrome, dysmenorrhoea, post-menopausal osteoporosis and migraine. Most of the evidence comes from poorly conducted trials, and magnesium does not appear to be very useful as a dietary supplement. Intravenous magnesium may reduce mortality in patients with acute myocardial infarction, but there is no justification for using oral magnesium as a dietary supplement for the prevention of heart attacks.

Selenium

Selenium is an anti-oxidant mineral which acts as a scavenger of free radicals. Like vitamins A, C, E and beta-carotene, selenium has been advocated for the prevention of cancer and there is some evidence that it reduces the risk of prostate cancer. It is also promoted for the prevention of coronary heart disease and for delaying the ageing process.

Zinc

Zinc supplements have been advocated for the treatment and prevention of colds and skin disorders such as acne, eczema and psoriasis, but evidence for a beneficial effect in these conditions is inconclusive. Patients with impaired wound healing may have low zinc levels, and for such people a supplement might be useful.

Toxicity of vitamins and minerals

When giving advice on the use of dietary supplements, one of the most important roles for the pharmacist is to give appropriate warnings about toxicity and overdosage. Safe levels for daily self-supplementation are given in Table 25.3. Details of interactions between dietary supplements and drugs can be found in Chapter 26.

Table 25.3   Safe levels for daily self-supplementation.

Vitamin or mineral	Upper safe level for daily self-supplementation
Vitamin A (µg)	2,300
Vitamin D (µg)	10
Vitamin E (mg)	800
Niacin (mg)	450
Nicotinic acid (mg)	150
Pyridoxine (mg)	50
Folic acid (µg)	400
Vitamin C (mg)	2,000
Calcium (mg)	1,500
Magnesium (mg)	350
Copper (mg)	5
Chromium (µg)	200
Iodine (µg)	500
Iron (mg)	15
Selenium (µg)	200
Zinc (mg)	15

Single vitamin and mineral preparations are best avoided for two reasons. First, many nutrients are absorbed by similar transport processes in the gut and an excess of one vitamin or mineral might prejudice the absorption of another. Secondly, one vitamin is often required for the metabolism of another. Riboflavin, for example, is involved in the metabolism of pyridoxine, so a large dose of pyridoxine could cause a deficiency of riboflavin.

Vitamin A

Toxic effects of vitamin A are well known in both children and adults. Acute poisoning may occur after a single dose of 30 mg (1 000 000 IU) of vitamin A.

If taken over several months, doses of 7.5–15 mg (25 000–50 000 IU) can cause toxicity and it is not difficult to obtain this amount of vitamin A from some of the available dietary supplements. Symptoms include dry, itchy skin, cracked lips and liver damage. Large doses of vitamin A are teratogenic so vitamin A supplements containing more than the RDA should be avoided by women who are pregnant or who are likely to become so (see Chapter 15).

Beta-carotene is generally non-toxic. Excessive intake of supplements or of carrot juice, which contains a high concentration of beta-carotene, may cause an orange coloration of the skin. This condition can be distinguished from jaundice because the sclera remain uncoloured. Skin coloration disappears within a few days of stopping beta-carotene.

Vitamin B$_6$

In high dosage, Vitamin B$_6$ has an adverse effect on the peripheral nervous system, and may cause peripheral sensory neuropathy. However, in doses up to 50 mg daily it appears safe and symptoms of toxicity – which are generally reversible – have not frequently been demonstrated in doses of less than 200–500 mg daily.

Niacin

The majority of people who take large doses of nicotinic acid will experience skin flushing. In doses exceeding 500 mg a day, nicotinic acid has been associated with liver damage. Most, but not all, the formulations have been sustained release products. The critical factor could be the dose or the formulation or both. In high dosage, nicotinic acid may aggravate peptic ulcers and alter glucose tolerance.

Nitocinamide alone, which is the form found in most dietary supplements, does not appear to produce any of these adverse effects.

Folic acid

Folic acid is not generally toxic, even in large doses, but care should be taken not to exceed the recommended doses in pregnancy (see Chapter 15). Folic acid should not be used in cases of undiagnosed megaloblastic anaemia because it may precipitate neuropathy (see Chapter 10).

Vitamin C

High doses of vitamin C are relatively harmless, but may cause diarrhoea. Individuals who stop taking vitamin C have an increased risk of rebound scurvy. In doses of 4 to 8 g a day, vitamin C may cause renal oxalate stones but there is little evidence for this. However, patients with renal impairment should avoid high doses of vitamin C.

People who take large amounts of vitamin C show a false positive reaction on urine-glucose testing with Clinitest. This is because vitamin C is a reducing agent like glucose. On the other hand, a false negative reaction may occur on testing with Clinistix and with any blood glucose test kit. This is because vitamin C inhibits the reaction which gives the colour.

Vitamin D

Intakes of vitamin D exceeding 500 µg (20 000 IU) are toxic and may lead to the development of hypercalcaemia with its associated symptoms of muscle weakness, bone pain, gastrointestinal disturbances and headaches. Individual tolerance to vitamin D varies considerably, and infants and children are generally more susceptible to its toxic effects than adults. Caution should be exercised in the use of paediatric vitamin drops. Overdosage of both vitamins A and D may occur if a dose of 5 ml is given accidentally instead of 5 drops. Vitamin D in doses exceeding 10 µg (400 IU)/day should be avoided by mothers who are breast feeding because of the risk of hypercalcaemia in the infant.

Vitamin E

There appears to be little risk of toxicity with even quite large doses of vitamin E (100–800 IU). Doses over 1000 IU may cause gastrointestinal disturbances.

Calcium

Unless a patient has renal impairment or a history of kidney stones, calcium supplements are generally safe and there is no harm in daily doses from supplements of up to 1 g of elemental calcium.

Iron

Iron salts commonly causes gastrointestinal symptoms even in usual doses. In doses exceeding 20 mg/kg, more toxic symptoms, such as circulatory failure and liver damage, may occur. In a child weighing 20 kg this is equivalent to only seven ferrous sulphate tablets. Adults should be warned about the dangers of leaving iron tablets around when there are children in the house.

Magnesium

Magnesium supplements are not likely to be harmful except in patients with renal failure who should not take large doses. Magnesium salts also have a laxative effect.

Selenium

Selenium is toxic in high doses. Side effects include hair loss, gastrointestinal disturbances and discoloration of the nails. However, the doses of selenium recommended by the manufacturers of most of the dietary supplements are quite safe. As a guide, daily doses over 1 mg should be avoided.

Zinc

Zinc is relatively non-toxic if taken orally, the only immediate adverse effects being nausea and dyspepsia. However high doses of zinc (> 300 mg a day) may decrease levels of HDL cholesterol; high levels of HDL are thought to be protective against heart disease.

Zinc competes with both copper and iron for absorption in the intestine and even moderate doses of zinc (20 mg a day) may impair the absorption of copper and iron. Zinc absorption is reduced by oral iron. For this reason, single mineral supplements should not be recommended except in cases of diagnosed deficiency.

Health supplements

Fish liver oils and fish oils

Fish liver oils have traditionally been used because they are a rich source of vitamins A and D but they are also rich in polyunsaturated fatty acids, particularly eicosapentaenoic acid (EPA) and docosahexaenoic acid (DHA). EPA and DHA can be synthesised in the body, but their direct consumption appears to have a distinct therapeutic effect.

The consumption of these fatty acids lowers the level of serum triglycerides. A fish oil concentrate, Maxepa (Seven Seas), is a licensed medicine for the treatment of hypertriglyceridaemia. EPA and DHA also appear to influence blood clotting by reducing the adhesiveness of platelets so they may reduce the tendency to thrombosis.

EPA and DHA also have anti-inflammatory effects. Some clinical trials have shown that fish oils help to alleviate inflammatory skin conditions such as psoriasis and eczema. Patients with rheumatoid arthritis may also find fish oil supplements helpful.

Many people dislike the taste of cod liver oil and for this reason they often prefer a capsule formulation. Whilst cod liver capsules are a useful source of vitamins A and D, they contain much less EPA and DHA than the liquid (see Table 25.4).

Excessive intakes of fish liver oils can lead to vitamin A and D toxicity. Cod liver oil supplements do not generally pose a hazard in this respect because a 10 ml dose contains no more than the RNI of each vitamin. However, the practice of taking tablespoons of cod liver oil should certainly be discouraged. Cod liver oil is also rich in energy: 10 ml provides about 336 kJ (80 kcal). Halibut liver oils and shark liver oils contain much higher concentrations of vitamins A and D than cod liver oil and should be used with caution.

Fish liver oils should be distinguished from fish flesh oils. Oils from the

Table 25.4 Amounts of eicosapentaenoic acid (EPA) and docosahexanoic acid (DHA) in some dietary supplements.

Supplement	EPA/DHA
Capsules (mg/capsule)	
Sanatogen (Roche)	
High strength cod liver oil	158
Super cod liver oil one-a-day	103
Seven Seas	
High strength one-a-day	180
Extra high strength one-a-day	360
One-a-day pure cod liver oil	84
Pure cod liver oil	100
Pulse	107
Pulse high strength triomega	260
Liquids (mg/10 ml)	
Sanatogen (Roche)	
Super cod liver oil	1800
Seven Seas	
Pure cod liver oil	1564
Pure cod liver oil lemon flavour	1488
Orange syrup and cod liver oil	476
High strength pure cod liver oil	2240
Extra high strength pure cod liver oil	1800
Lemon flavour cod liver oil with evening primrose oil	1405

flesh of the fish rather than the liver are low in vitamins A and D but rich in EPA and DHA.

Gamma-linolenic acid

Gamma-linolenic acid is a polyunsaturated fatty acid of the n-6 series. It is synthesised in the body from dietary linoleic acid, but its direct consumption does appear to have different effects from those obtained by consuming linoleic acid.

Evening primrose oil, borage seed oil (also known as starflower oil), blackcurrant seed oil and oil of Javanicus are sold as sources of supplementary gamma-linolenic acid (see Table 25.5).

It is prescribable in the UK (as gamolenic rather than gamma-linolenic acid) for the symptomatic relief of eczema (Epogam) and breast pain (Efamast). Claims for a beneficial effect in other conditions, such as premenstrual tension, multiple sclerosis, asthma and rheumatoid arthritis, have not been substantiated.

Side-effects are uncommon but headaches and nausea occasionally occur; these symptoms may be improved by taking the supplement with food. Gamma-linolenic acid appears to increase the risk of epilepsy particularly in patients taking phenothiazines (see Chapter 26).

Table 25.5   Amounts of gamma-linolenic acid (GLA) in some dietary supplements.

Supplement	GLA
Capsules (mg/capsule)	
Efamol products (Britannia)	
Efamol	40
Efamol PMP	40
Efamol + Safflower & Linseed Oils	20
Floresse (Roche)	
Starflower Oil 250 mg	57
Starflower Oil 500 mg	115
Starflower Oil 1000 mg	230
Seven Seas	
Evening Primrose Oil Pure 500 mg	37
Evening Primrose Oil Pure 1000 mg	74
Evening Primrose Oil plus Starflower Oil 500 mg	65
Evening Primrose Oil plus Starflower Oil 1000 mg	130
Liquids (mg/10 ml)	
Seven Seas	
Cod Liver Oil and Evening Primrose Oil	33

Garlic

Garlic has been used medicinally for centuries and is widely promoted for colds and coughs. There is some evidence that garlic has beneficial effects in lowering serum cholesterol and in reducing platelet aggregation although most trials to date have been of poor quality. Garlic may also be protective against the development of certain cancers, and it appears to have some antibacterial and antifungal activity.

Ginseng

Ginseng has been used by the Chinese for over 2000 years and is available commercially as roots, powdered roots, tablets, capsules, teas, oils and extracts. It contains complex mixtures of saponins called ginsenosides. Ginseng is claimed to act as a tonic that restors, maintains and builds up the whole body.

There is quite a high incidence of side-effects with ginseng. Doses as low as 3 g may cause diarrhoea, skin rashes, sleeplessness, nervousness, euphoria, hypertension and oedema. Ginseng appears to have oestrogenic effects and should certainly be avoided by women during pregnancy and at the time of the menopause.

Glucosamine

Glucosamine is a natural substance found in various mucopolysaccharides, mucoproteins and chitin. As a supplement, it is synthetically manufactured, and it is thought to be useful in patients with osteoarthritis and other joint disorders. Several trials have shown that it can improve symptoms of osteoarthritis and it appears to work by rebuilding damaged cartilage. However, all the trials so far have contained major study flaws and long-term, well designed controlled studies are needed before glucosamine's role in the treatment of osteoarthritis can be clarified.

Green lipped mussel

Green lipped mussel is promoted as a natural treatment for arthritis and this is very attractive to people who cannot tolerate the side-effects of non-steroidal anti-inflammatory drugs (NSAIDs). Whilst green lipped mussel appears to contain a weak anti-inflammatory substance, there is little evidence that it works. It appears to be relatively safe, and reported side-effects are mainly limited to gastrointestinal disturbances.

Kelp

Kelp is a preparation obtained from seaweed which is promoted for general health and well-being. It is rich in iodine but iodine content is not always declared on the label. Supplemental iodine may lead to disturbances of the thyroid gland, and kelp should be avoided by patients with thyroid disorders.

Pharmacists should be aware of the potential for dangerous contaminants in kelp preparations. Kelp can concentrate heavy metals, and products may contain substantial amounts of arsenic.

Royal jelly

Royal jelly has become an extremely popular dietary supplement in recent years and is promoted mainly for its rejuvenating properties. While it does contain some vitamins and minerals, these are in very small amounts and far greater concentrations of nutrients can be found in most normal foods. It seems likely that any reported benefits of royal jelly are due to its placebo effect. It does, however, appear to be safe except in patients with asthma; two deaths have been reported from royal jelly consumption in Australia.

The role of the pharmacist

When asked about dietary supplements pharmacists should always ask questions about the diet and emphasise the importance of healthy eating (see Chapter 3). A dietary supplement does not turn an unhealthy diet into a healthy one.

If appropriate, questions may be asked about the perceived need for the supplement and any expectations assessed. An awareness of the groups of people who could benefit from supplements is important. It is vital to establish whether other medicines (including other dietary supplements) are being taken or whether the person is pregnant or suffers from any disease.

The safest supplements are those which contain a wide variety of vitamins and minerals in quantities that do not exceed the RNI (or RDA). Advice about appropriate dosage and warnings about overdosage should always be given. The list of ingredients should be checked for substances that the individual may want to avoid (e.g. gluten, gelatin or lactose).

The use of single vitamins and minerals should be discouraged. If these are required they should be prescribed by the doctor.

Further reading

Bender, A.E. (1985) *Health or Hoax*. Elvedon Press, Reading.

Ministry of Agriculture, Fisheries and Food, Department of Health (1991) Dietary Supplements and Health Foods. Report of a working group. MAFF Publications, London.

National Dairy Council (1988) Vitamins, Minerals and Health. Fact File No 3. The National Dairy Council, London.

National Dairy Council (1992) Calcium and Health. Fact File No 1. The National Dairy Council, London.

Chapter 26
Drug–Nutrient Interactions

Drugs and nutrients share several characteristics, including similar sites of absorption in the intestine, the ability to alter physiological processes and the capacity to cause toxicity in high doses. In the same way as a drug can interact with another drug, so a drug may interact with a nutrient.

Drugs can interact with food and nutrients in several ways. They can cause nutrient deficiencies and changes in appetite, taste and body weight. Some can influence cholesterol and glucose metabolism. Drug absorption and metabolism can be altered by dietary supplements and by the presence of absence of food. Changes in body weight may also influence drug metabolism. Certain foods can cause toxic reactions with drugs (e.g. monoamine oxidase inhibitors and cheese) and alcohol increases the sedative effects of several drugs.

Clinical importance

Drug–nutrient interactions may result in reduction of drug efficacy, or even in complete failure of drug therapy, although this is quite rare. Many drug–nutrient interactions are fairly harmless, since most drugs are designed to produce blood levels well above those required for therapeutic efficacy. So, if some aspect of diet reduces the blood levels of a drug, this may not prejudice its clinical effects. Drugs with a small therapeutic range (e.g. phenytoin and theophylline) and those drugs whose dosage needs careful control (e.g. anticoagulants) are those where drug–nutrient interactions are likely to be most important.

The potential for drug–nutrient interactions is increased if drugs are taken at meal times or if patients make major changes to the composition of their diet, lose or gain a great deal of weight in a short time or take large doses of dietary supplements. If patients are already at risk of nutrient deficiency because of poor diet or disease, the administration of drugs may increase the risk further.

Patients at risk

The severity of interactions differs from one patient to another and some groups of patients are at particular risk.

Infants and children are at particular risk because of the relative ineffi-ciency of the drug-metabolising enzymes and poorly developed kidney function.

Patients on multiple or long-term drug therapy (e.g. the elderly patient with diabetes mellitus, arthritis or cardiovascular disease) are more at risk than patients on a short course of antibiotics.

The risk of drug–nutrient interactions is increased in patients who are already malnourished because of a poor diet (e.g. alcoholics and those on low incomes) and in those with diseases which may themselves lead to nutrient deficiencies (e.g. coeliac disease, renal and liver failure). The risk is also greater in patients who have increased nutritional requirements (e.g. those with cancer or severe burns).

Care should always be taken with drug regimens for patients on enteral and parenteral nutrition because of the possibility of an interaction between the feed and the drug (see p. 249).

The influence of drugs on nutrition

Drugs may affect nutrient intake, absorption, metabolism and excretion. They may also lead to changes in glucose and cholesterol metabolism, and in tissue function and body weight.

Nutrient intake

The administration of drugs may affect nutrient intake by causing gastro-intestinal disturbances or by altering appetite and taste. There are a great number of drugs which can cause nausea and vomiting as a side-effect, and any of these drugs could affect a patient's desire to eat.

Appetite

Drugs which lead to changes in appetite are shown in Tables 26.1 and 26.2. Drugs which reduce appetite may result in poor nutrition and weight loss, whilst drugs which increase appetite may lead to weight gain. If a patient complains of poor appetite, pharmacists should be aware that a prescribed drug could be one of the causes. A change of drug may be warranted.

Taste

Drugs may also lead to alterations in taste (see Table 26.3) and some of these changes can be unpleasant. Again, the patient's desire to eat may be reduced.

Nutrient absorption

Drugs may affect nutrient absorption by changing gastrointestinal motility or pH, or by forming insoluble complexes with dietary components.

Table 26.1 Drugs reported to reduce appetite.

Digoxin	Lithium
Fluoexitine	Metformin
Levodopa	Nitrofurantoin

Table 26.2 Drugs reported to increase appetite.

Cyproheptadine	Sodium valproate
Monoamine oxidase inhibitors	Tricyclic antidepressants
Pizotifen	(particularly amitriptyline)

Table 26.3 Drugs reported to affect taste.

ACE inhibitors	Metronidazole
Amiodarone (metallic taste)	Nedocromil
Aztreonam	Penicillamine
Baclofcn	4-Quinoloncs
Calcitonin	Propafenone
Disodium etidronate	

Gastrointestinal motility

Gastrointestinal motility can be altered by drugs such as laxatives, meto-clopramide and antimuscarinics. Antimuscarinics reduce motility while laxatives and metoclopramide increase it.

A reduction in motility is very unlikely to affect nutrient absorption, but an increase in motility may reduce absorption of nutrients. Stimulant laxatives (e.g. bisacodyl and senna) can lead to depletion of minerals, and liquid paraffin causes malabsorption of fat-soluble vitamins. This is one of the reasons why laxatives should not be used for long periods of time.

Gastrointestinal pH

Some nutrients are preferentially absorbed in one form. For example, iron is absorbed in the ferrous (Fe^{2+}) form while the ferric (Fe^{3+}) form is insoluble and poorly absorbed. If the pH of the intestine increases, the ferric form of iron is precipitated.

The administration of any drug which increases the pH in the intestine will lead to poor iron absorption. This is why antacids should never be administered with oral iron preparations. This situation can easily arise in pregnancy. If a pregnant woman needs to take both antacids and iron, she should be advised to separate the doses of the two products by at least 2 hours.

Insoluble complexes

Minerals such as iron and zinc form insoluble complexes with drugs such as tetracyclines and 4-quinolones. This leads not only to poor absorption of the mineral, but also to poor absorption of the drug. Antacids tend to bind iron in the gut and this may be a particular problem for pregnant women, some of whom will be obtaining iron on prescription and antacids over the counter. If patients need to take these incompatible preparations, they should separate the doses by at least 2 hours.

Penicillamine is a drug used to chelate excess copper in the treatment of Wilson's disease (see Chapter 12). Penicillamine also chelates iron and zinc, but supplements should not be used. This is because the drug could chelate iron and zinc in preference to copper, resulting in failure of the treatment.

The absorption of the fat-soluble vitamins (A, D, E, K) and folic acid is reduced by the lipid-lowering drugs cholestyramine and colestipol. These drugs often increase the tendency to bleed which is associated with malabsorption of vitamin K. Supplements of all these vitamins may be prescribed if the patient is on long-term treatment with either of these drugs.

Nutrient metabolism

Some drugs have antivitamin effects and are known as vitamin antagonists. These include isoniazid, menoamine oxidase inhibitors, methotrexate, phenobarbitone, phenytoin, primidone, pyrimethamine, sulphasalazine and trimethoprim.

Isoniazid and monoamine oxidase inhibitors affect pyridoxine metabolism and may cause peripheral neuritis. The risk of this seems to be greatest with isoniazid, so that pyridoxine supplements are often prescribed with this drug.

Phenytoin and other anticonvulsants may interfere with vitamin D metabolism by inducing the drug-metabolising enzymes in the liver. In the absence of an adequate dietary intake of vitamin D or where there is minimal exposure to sunlight, osteomalacia or rickets may occur. It is important that patients who avoid direct sunlight either because they are housebound, or because they cover most of their skin with clothing, be encouraged to consume foods rich in vitamin D (see Appendix 5). Children prescribed long-term anticonvulsant therapy should take a vitamin D supplement.

Phenobarbitone, phenytoin, primidone, pyrimethamine, sulphasalazine and trimethoprim are folic acid antagonists. Caution should be exercised in the use of these drugs in patients in whom folic acid may be deficient, and blood counts should be checked regularly because of the risk of megaloblastic anaemia. Women taking anticonvulsants during pregnancy or when planning a pregnancy should be advised of the risks of producing an infant with a neural tube defect (see Chapter 15) and a folic acid supplement should be prescribed by the doctor.

Oral contraceptives have been reported to alter the metabolism of several vitamins including vitamin A, vitamin C, vitamin B_6, vitamin B_{12} and folic acid. However, these effects seem to be very variable and may not be as important now that the amount of oestrogen in the formulations has been reduced. There is little justification for women on oral contraceptives taking multivitamin preparations.

Nutrient excretion

Drugs may affect the excretion of minerals by inhibiting or promoting their reabsorption in the kidney tubule. Corticosteroids and carbenoxolone tend to cause retention of sodium and depletion of potassium. Diuretics increase the excretion of sodium, potassium and magnesium. Thiazides reduce the excretion of calcium.

Diuretic therapy is associated with a fall in serum potassium concentration but marked hypokalaemia is rare. The risk of hypokalaemia is minimal with low doses of thiazides (e.g. 2.5 mg of bendrofluazide daily); it is greater with high doses of diuretics and if other potassium-depleting drugs, such as corticosteroids and laxatives, are prescribed at the same time. Hypokalaemia is of most concern in patients taking digoxin, amiodarone, disopyramide and flecainide because of the risk of cardiac arrhythmias.

Prevention of hypokalaemia is best achieved by using the lowest dose of diuretic which produces the desired therapeutic effect. High potassium diets are often recommended, but to achieve a significant increase in serum potassium requires huge and impractical amounts of potassium-rich foods. If potassium conservation is considered to be necessary, a potassium-sparing diuretic (e.g. amiloride or triamterene) should be used in preference to a potassium supplement.

Glucose metabolism

Oral antidiabetic drugs are intended to reduce blood glucose levels, but many other drugs alter blood glucose levels as a side-effect. Clearly, the greatest risk with these drugs is in patients with diabetes mellitus.

Drugs which may induce hyperglycaemia include the corticosteroids, tricyclic antidepressants and both the loop and thiazide diuretics. Sympathomimetics found in several OTC preparations may also raise blood glucose levels and should not be sold to patients with diabetes.

The main group of drugs which lower blood glucose levels is the beta-blockers but this effect is usually very small.

Cholesterol metabolism

Obviously, all the lipid-lowering drugs are designed to reduce blood cholesterol levels. However, there has been some concern about the loop and thiazide diuretics which appear to increase serum cholesterol levels, but these effects appear to be minimal.

Oral contraceptives produce small increases in blood cholesterol, but whether these changes are clinically important is not known.

Tissue function

Drugs may affect tissue function and induce a nutritional deficiency. For example, NSAIDs can cause bleeding from the gastrointestinal tract. If gastrointestinal bleeding is prolonged, this could result in anaemia.

Body weight

The administration of drugs may lead to either weight loss or weight gain. Appetite suppressants and thyroid hormones are the main examples of drugs which lead to weight loss, but drugs which reduce appetite (see Table 26.1) may also result in loss of weight.

Other drugs may cause weight gain (see Table 26.4). Some of these, e.g. carbenoxolone and minoxidil, induce oedema, and weight gain is therefore due to fluid retention rather than gain in body fat.

If weight loss or gain is a problem, it may be worth discussing an alternative drug with the prescriber.

Table 26.4   Drugs reported to increase body weight.

Astemizole	Monoamine oxidase inhibitors
Carbenoxolone	Oral contraceptives
Lithium	Phenothiazines
Indoramin	Vigabatrin
Minoxidil	

Interactions between drugs and dietary supplements

The popularity of dietary supplements is increasing, and pharmacists should be aware that some supplements are contraindicated when certain drugs are taken. Before selling a supplement pharmacists should always ask if the person is taking other medicines.

Large doses of vitamin E (> 400 IU) potentiate the effects of anticoagulants and may cause bleeding in patients taking these drugs.

In contrast, vitamin K tends to antagonise the effects of anticoagulants. Anticoagulants compete with vitamin K to reduce the production of blood-clotting factors. If the supply of vitamin K is boosted by abnormally large intakes, the production of blood-clotting factors is favoured and the effects of the anticoagulant are reduced.

Large doses of vitamin B_6 reduce the blood levels of phenobarbitone and phenytoin. Small doses are unlikely to cause problems, and if patients are taking multivitamin supplements they should be warned not to exceed a daily dose of 10 mg of vitamin B_6.

Doses of vitamin B_6 as low as 5–10 mg can reduce or abolish the effects of levodopa. Patients must be warned not to take any vitamin B_6 supplements with levodopa. Dietary intake need not be adjusted; this is impractical, and in any case pyridoxine is required for the transformation of levodopa to dopamine. It is only when pyridoxine is in excess that wasteful transformation of levodopa occurs outside the brain and the drug does not reach its site of action. This interaction can be avoided by prescribing a compound preparation containing levodopa with a dopa-decarboxylase inhibitor (e.g. co-beneldopa or co-careldopa).

Iron binds several drugs in the gastrointestinal tract with a consequent reduction in the absorption of both the drug and iron. Chelation of levodopa by iron can lead to reduced control of Parkinson's disease.

Both iron and zinc form insoluble complexes with several antibacterials, including the tetracyclines and some of the 4-quinolones (e.g. ciprofloxacin, norfloxacin and ofloxacin), and with penicillamine. Calcium reduces the absorption of tetracyclines.

Because drug absorption is often reduced by more than one mineral, it is wise to avoid taking preparations containing any minerals with the drugs mentioned in this section. If, for any reason, they cannot be avoided, doses should always be separated by at least 2 hours.

Potassium supplements (including salt substitutes) should be avoided by patients taking ACE inhibitors (e.g. captopril), potassium-sparing diuretics (e.g. amiloride) and cyclosporin because of a risk of severe hyperkalaemia which may be life threatening.

Calcium supplements are best avoided by patients taking thiazide diuretics because these drugs reduce the excretion of calcium.

Fish liver oils (e.g. cod liver oil) and fish oils contain the fatty acids eicosapentaenoic acid and docosahexaenoic acid, which may alter the coagulability of the blood. These supplements are best avoided by patients taking anticoagulants.

Evening primrose oil appears to increase the risk of epileptic side-effects in patients taking phenothiazines. Supplements should be avoided by anyone taking these drugs and by anyone with epilepsy or a history of the disease.

Interactions between drugs and enteral and parenteral feeds

Drugs are often required by patients on enteral or parenteral feeds, but incompatibilities can occur. Drugs should not normally be given at the same time as an enteral feed, and should never be administered down intravenous feeding lines.

Where drug–feed incompatibilities are recognised, it is advisable, if possible, to leave a gap of 2 hours between the end of the feed and the administration of the drug. The feeding tube should be thoroughly washed before and after the drug is given.

Antacids can interact with enteral feeds to produce an obstructive plug in the oesophagus. A marked reduction in phenytoin absorption has been reported with enteral feeds. The bioavailability of theophylline may be reduced in patients who receive either enteral or parenteral feeds which are high in protein.

Many enteral feeds contain vitamin K which may interfere with the metabolism of anticoagulants. The ingestion of as little as 50 µg of vitamin K may lead to changes in prothrombin time. The significance of an interaction between warfarin and vitamin K depends on how much of the enteral feed is consumed.

Several enteral feeds contain more than 30 µg of vitamin K in 4.2 MJ (1000 kcal), but formulations keep changing and labels should always be checked. Prescribers should be alerted to the possibility of this interaction and advised to check prothrombin times regularly. Doses of anticoagulants may need altering, both while the patient is receiving the enteral feeds and also when they are discontinued.

The influence of food on drug therapy

Pharmacists will be familiar with patients asking whether they should take their medicines before or after food. The timing of drug administration in relation to meals can be important, but what is often overlooked is the importance of using snacks or mealtimes as a means of aiding compliance.

Breakfast, lunch, dinner and supper tend to be such familiar routines that they can be used as 'memory joggers' to remind patients to take their medicines. Waking up an hour before breakfast or stopping the car on the way home from work to take a tablet can be very inconvenient, and may mean that the dose is missed completely if the patient thinks that the medicine must be taken an hour before food.

Drug absorption

The presence of food in the gastrointestinal tract alters gastric emptying rate and stimulates the secretion of digestive juices and enzymes, effects which can influence both the rate and the extent of drug absorption.

Gastric emptying rate

Changes in gastric emptying rate can alter either the rate or the extent of drug absorption or both. Alteration in the rate of drug absorption tends to be less important than change in the total amount absorbed.

Solid food, particularly food rich in fat or non-starch polysaccharides (NSP), delays gastric emptying whereas fluid speeds it up. Food will therefore delay the arrival of an orally administered drug in the duodenum. Because most drugs are optimally absorbed in the small intestine, the presence of food will reduce the rate of drug absorption and therefore delay the onset of therapeutic action.

In general, the most rapid therapeutic response can be achieved by taking a drug with plenty of fluid on an empty stomach. This is particularly important where an immediate therapeutic response is required, such as when an analgesic is taken to relieve a headache or a sedative to induce sleep. On the other hand, many analgesics cause gastrointestinal irritation which can often be avoided if the drug is taken with food. Delay in drug absorption is likely to be more important where therapeutic efficacy is dependent on the maintenance of consistent blood levels of the drug. This has traditionally been considered to be important with antibiotics, but it may not be quite as crucial as was once believed.

Gastrointestinal secretions

Food, particularly if it contains a large quantity of fat, promotes the secretion of the pancreatic enzymes and bile. Whilst the pancreatic enzymes have a very limited effect on drug absorption, bile may have a significant effect. Bile salts are surface-active agents and can increase the dissolution of some drugs with a consequent enhancement in absorption. The improvement in absorption of griseofulvin with a fatty meal is probably due to the solubilising effect of bile salts secreted in response to the ingestion of fat.

Drug metabolism

Drugs are metabolised in the liver and food can affect this in several ways. Food causes an increase in blood flow to the liver and this increases the rate at which drugs pass through the liver into the systemic circulation. If a drug is particularly susceptible to degradation in the liver (e.g. labetalol), a larger proportion of the drug will pass intact into the systemic circulation.

Certain types of food stimulate the drug metabolising enzymes. Large amounts of green vegetables, such as broccoli, Brussels sprouts, spinach and cabbage, appear to reduce the anticoagulant effect of warfarin. These vegetables contain substances known as indoles which stimulate the drug-metabolising enzymes and increase the rate at which warfarin is metabolised and eliminated from the body. Green vegetables also contain large concentrations of vitamin K which has a separate effect on the metabolism of warfarin (see p. 248).

There have also been some rare reports of large quantities of ice cream (> 1 litre) reducing the anticoagulant effects of warfarin. The reasons for this are not known.

Grapefruit juice inactivates the main intestinal drug-metabolising enzyme (CYP 3A4) and so increases the absorption of some calcium-channel blockers (e.g. felodipine, isradipine, lacidipine, lercanidipine, nimodipine, nicardipine, nifedipine and nisoldipine) and HIV-1 protease inhibitors. However, grapefruit juice appears to antagonise the absorption of some drugs such as cyclosporine, digoxin, fexofenadine, losartan and vinblastine. The juice activates the efflux pump, P-glycoprotein, which ejects drug molecules out of the gut wall back into the intestine. Patients taking any of these drugs should be careful about drinking grapefruit juice, and the juice is best taken about two hours before taking the drugs.

In addition, grapefruit juice may increase plasma concentration of terfenadine and cause cardiotoxicity; grapefruit juice is best avoided when taking this drug.

The influence of body weight on drug therapy

The amount of body fat may alter drug distribution in the tissues. If body fat content increases, fat-soluble drugs (e.g. benzodiazepines, phenytoin) will be drawn preferentially into the adipose tissue rather than to the site of action. This could lead to a reduction in the clinical effectiveness of the drug. On the other hand, if a patient loses body fat, a lipid-soluble drug may become more therapeutically active.

Everybody should be discouraged from going on 'crash' diets, but this is particularly important for a patient on long-term drug therapy. If weight loss is necessary, it should be achieved gradually. Pharmacists should be alert for any adverse drug effects or any worsening of symptom control in patients who have lost or gained a great deal of weight over a short period of time. It may be worth discussing an adjustment in drug dosage with the prescriber.

The influence of malnutrition on drug therapy

Community pharmacists will rarely see malnourished patients, but they should be aware of the differences which severe malnutrition can make to drug therapy. If a patient is severely malnourished (e.g. Body Mass Index: weight/height^2 below 20), there may be some loss of absorptive capacity in the intestine. Loss of kidney function could lead to drug toxicity.

Severe malnutrition is likely to lead to reduced activity of the drug metabolising enzymes. This may result in drug toxicity and a need to reduce the dose. The dose may then need to be gradually increased as the patient's condition improves.

Most drugs are bound to plasma proteins, particularly to the albumin fraction, but it is the unbound portion of the drug which is therapeutically active. Severe malnutrition causes a fall in plasma albumin and can therefore increase the proportion of a drug which is free to reach the site of action. This only produces a detectable effect if the drug is highly protein bound (e.g. warfarin), and any increase in clinical effect may only be transient because an increase in the concentration of unbound drug results in an increase in its elimination.

Drug-induced reactions to food

Pharmacists will be very familiar with the possibility of drug-induced reactions to components of food (Table 26.5), particularly with the reaction between tyramine and monoamine oxidase inhibitors which is potentially the most serious. A less frequent reaction is that between histamine and isoniazid. Whether or not these reactions occur, and also how severe the reaction is, depend on the drug dose, the frequency of drug administration, the concentration of the offending substance in the food and the quantity of food consumed.

Tyramine

The reaction between tyramine and MAOIs is serious and can be fatal. Symptoms include a violent headache, a pounding heart, sweating, nausea and vomiting, and there is a rapid rise in blood pressure. All the MAOIs (i.e. phenelzine, tranylcypromine and isocarboxazid) have been implicated.

Tyramine is formed in foods by the bacterial degradation of milk and other proteins. Normally, any ingested tyramine is rapidly metabolised by the enzyme monoamine oxidase in the intestinal wall and the liver, but when a patient takes MAOIs the enzyme is destroyed and any ingested tyramine passes freely into the tissues where it increases the release of noradrenaline. The release of nonadrenaline causes a rapid rise in blood pressure. As little as 6 mg of tyramine can produce a rise in blood pressure and 10–25 mg may result in a serious reaction.

It is extremely difficult to predict the tyramine content of food. The tyramine content of cheeses can vary between 0 and 2 mg/g. An old and mature cheese may sometimes contain less tyramine than a mild-tasting variety. The tyramine content of a single cheese can even vary significantly between the centre and the rind. Stilton cheese generally contains large amounts which may exceed 2 mg/g, but Cheddar cheese may also contain significant amounts. Brie and Camembert often contain only small amounts of tyramine (0.1 mg/g), but should not be eaten by patients taking MAOIs. Because of this unpredictable variation in tyramine content all cheese are prohibited to patients taking MAOIs, the only exceptions being plain cottage cheese and plain cream cheese which are likely to be safe.

All yeast extracts contain considerable quantities of tyramine. Marmite contains the greatest amounts, but Bovril, Oxo and vegetarian yeast spreads should also be avoided. Twiglets also contain significant amounts of yeast extract so should also be avoided.

Brewer's yeast tablets are also prohibited and several other dietary supplements, particularly those containing vitamin B, may well contain yeast extract. However, several dietary supplements are yeast free so labels should be checked.

Other foods which should be viewed with suspicion include pickled herrings, beef and chicken livers, fermented soy products (e.g. miso, tempeh and soy sauce), avocados, fermented milk products and fermented meats such as bolognas, salamis and pepperoni. Broad bean pods contain significant amounts of tyramine though the broad beans themselves are quite safe.

In general, patients on MAOIs should be advised to eat foods and definitely to avoid cheese, yeast extracts, pickled herrings and broad bean pods. Any meat, fish or poultry which may be going off should also be avoided.

Patients taking MAOIs should avoid alcohol and also alcohol-free wines and beers. Most alcoholic drinks are produced by a fermentation process and it is impossible to predict how much tyramine will be present. Whisky,

Table 26.5 Nutritional implications with drugs.

Drug	Nutritional implications	Advice
ACE inhibitors	Hyperkalaemia enhanced with potassium	Avoid preparations containing potassium, including salt substitutes (e.g. Losalt and Ruthmol)
Antacids	Magnesium trisilicate reduces absorption of oral iron	Separate doses of magnesium trisilicate from oral iron preparations by 2 hours
	Antacids react with enteral feeds to form an obstructive plug in the oesophagus	Separate doses of antacids and enteral feeds by 2 hours
Anticoagulants	Effects of warfarin may be enhanced and dicoumarol reduced by vitamin E	Avoid large doses of vitamin E (>100 IU)
	Effects of anticoagulants may be decreased or abolished by vitamin K	Avoid preparations containing vitamin K including enteral feeds and large amounts of green vegetables (e.g. broccoli, Brussels sprouts, spinach)
	Effects of anticoagulants may be enhanced by fish oils and fish liver oils	Avoid fish oils and fish liver oils
Anticonvulsants	Antagonise folic acid	Folic acid supplement[1]
	Plasma phenytoin and phenobarbitone concentration reduced by pyridoxine	Avoid large doses of pyridoxine (>200 mg)
	Phenytoin interferes with metabolism of vitamin D	Emphasise good sources of vitamin D in the diet or supplement[1]
Antifungals	Absorption of griseofulvin, itraconazole, ketoconazole, miconazole and tinidazole increased by food	Take with food
Calcium-channel blockers	Grapefruit juice increases serum levels of felodipine isradipine, lacidipine, lercanidipine, nicardipine, nifedipine, nimodipine and nisoldipine	Grapefruit juice is best taken at least 2 hours before these drugs
Cholestyramine & colestipol	Malabsorption of fat-soluble vitamins and folic acid	Supplements[1] of fat-soluble vitamins and folic acid
Cyclosporin	Hyperkalaemia enhanced with potassium	Avoid preparations containing potassium including salt substitutes (e.g. Losalt and Ruthmol)
Disodium etidronate	Absorption reduced by food, calcium, magnesium and iron	Avoid all food, milk and preparations containing calcium, magnesium and iron for at least 2 hours before and after drug administration
Diuretics	Risk of hyperkalaemia enhanced with potassium-sparing diuretics	Avoid preparations containing potassium and salt substitutes (e.g. Losalt and Ruthmol)

Cont.

Table 26.5 Cont.

Drug	Nutritional implications	Advice
Isoniazid	Possibility of toxic reaction with histamine	No dietary restrictions, but be aware of potential for reaction with cheese or fish
	Peripheral neuritis	Pyridoxine supplement[1]
Laxatives (stimulant)	Malabsorption of electrolytes	Avoid long-term use
Levodopa	Absorption of levodopa reduced by iron	Separate doses of levodopa and oral iron by at least 2 hours
	Effects reduced or abolished by pyridoxine	Avoid all supplements containing pyridoxine
Liquid paraffin	Malabsorption of fat-soluble vitamins	Avoid long-term use
Lithium	Plasma concentration reduced by increased intake of sodium and increased by reduced intake of sodium	Avoid any changes in salt intake or OTC medicines with a high sodium content
MAOIs	Toxic reaction with tyramine	Avoid cheese, pickled herring, broad bean pods, Bovril, Oxo, Marmite or yeast extract and stale food
	Peripheral neuritis	Pyridoxine supplement
Nitrofurantoin	Absorption increased by food	Take with food
Penicillamine	Absorption reduced by food and iron and zinc	Take half an hour before food and separate doses of penicillamine and oral iron and zinc by at least 2 hours
Phenothiazines	Epileptic side-effects increased with gamma-linolenic acid	Avoid gamma-linolenic acid (e.g. evening primrose oil)
Procarbazine	Mild MAOI effects with tyramine	No dietary restrictions
Pyrimethamine	Antagonises folic acid	Folic acid supplement[1]
4-Quinolones	Absorption of ciprofloxacin, norfloxacin and ofloxacin reduced by iron and zinc	Separate doses of 4-quinolones and oral iron or zinc by at least 2 hours
Sulphasalazine	Malabsorption of folic acid	Folic acid supplement[1]
Terfenadine	Grapefruit juice may increase plasma concentration of terfenadine and cause cardiotoxicity	Avoid grapefruit juice
Tetracyclines	Absorption reduced (except doxycycline and minocycline) by food (particularly dairy food)	Take 1 hour before food or on an empty stomach
	Absorption reduced by calcium, iron and zinc	Separate doses of tetracyclines and oral calcium, iron and zinc preparations by at least 2 hours

[1] Supplements should be prescribed by the doctor.

brandy and gin, which are produced by distillation, are unlikely to contain significant amounts of tyramine, but they do contain considerable amounts of alcohol and should not be drunk by patients on MAOIs because of the CNS depressant effect. Both low-alcohol and alcohol-free beers and wines contain significant amounts of tyramine and cannot be recommended as an alternative for patients taking MAOIs.

When MAOIs are withdrawn, the restriction on tyramine-containing foods and drinks should continue for 14 days to allow full recovery of the enzymes.

Histamine

Histamine reactions have been reported in patients who are taking isoniazid and eat certain types of fish, including tuna and sardines. These reactions are characterised by severe headache, facial flushing, dizziness, blurred vision and itching of the eyes. They occur because fish such as tuna, sardines, mackerel, pilchards and anchovies contain histamine. Mature cheeses may also contain significant amounts. Histamine is produced in these foods by the decarboxylation of the amino acid histidine. Histamine in food is normally inactivated by the enzyme histaminase, but isoniazid is a potent inhibitor of this enzyme. This means that histamine is absorbed unchanged and can cause unpleasant symptoms.

Because the incidence of the reaction is quite small, dietary restrictions are considered to be unnecessary. However, if any symptoms such as headache and flushing are reported by patients taking isoniazid, it is a wise precaution to ask about their diet.

Drugs and alcohol

Patients tend to be aware of the potential for adverse effects when alcohol is taken together with prescribed medicines, and frequently ask the pharmacist if drinking is allowed while taking a particular drug.

CNS depressants

Alcohol increases the sedative effects of all the CNS depressants such as barbiturates, benzodiazepines, antidepressants, tranquillisers, opioid analgesics, antinauseants and dextropropoxyphene. Increased sedation is also experienced with antihistamines, particularly the older ones such as chlorpheniramine and promethazine. It is much less of a problem with the newer compounds such as terfenadine and astemizole which do not cross the blood–brain barrier to any great extent. However, an interaction may occur, even with these newer antihistamines, if large amounts of alcohol are consumed.

Table 26.6   Some OTC medicines which contain alcohol.

Internal preparations
Bronalin Dry Cough
Dimotane Expectorant
Dimotane Co
Dimotane Co Paediatric
Hills Balsam Adult Expectorant
Labiton
Lemsip Night Time
Meltus Dry Cough
Robitussin
    Chesty Cough
    Chesty Cough with Congestion
    Dry Cough
    Junior for Persistent Coughs

External preparations
Alphosyl 2 in 1 Shampoo
Betadine Antiseptic Paint
Brush Off Cold Sore Treatment
Carlyderm Lotion
Ceanel Concentrate
Colsor Lotion
Cupal Cold Sore Lotion
DDD Medicated Lotion
Full Marks Lotion
Ionax Scrub
Ionil T
Panoxyl 5 and 10
Polytar Emollient and Liquid
Prioderm Lotion
Rapel Spray
Salactac Gel
Suleo-M
Suleo-C

Disulfiram

Disulfiram is used to treat alcohol dependence, and even small amounts of alcohol result in extremely toxic symptoms. Disulfiram inhibits acetaldehyde dehydrogenase, the enzyme responsible for the oxidation of acetaldehyde, the initial metabolite of alcohol. Alcohol consumption therefore results in acetaldehyde accumulation.

Symptoms include flushing of the face, throbbing headache, palpitations, nausea and vomiting. With larger doses of alcohol, arrhythmias, hypotension and collapse may follow. Even the smallest doses of alcohol included in several OTC medicines including external preparations (see Table 26.6) may be sufficient to cause a reaction. All alcohol should be avoided for 48 hours before the first dose and for 48 hours after the last dose.

Metronidazole

The disulfiram reaction may be experienced by patients taking metronidazole, nimorazole and tinidazole. Symptoms can occur not just with oral metronidazole preparations, but also with vaginal preparations.

Chlorpropamide

Chlorpropamide interacts with alcohol in about one-third of patients to produce a disulfiram-like reaction. Symptoms include flushing and tingling of the face and sometimes the neck, arms and eyes. Other oral hypoglycaemics do not produce this reaction.

Miscellaneous

Alcohol may potentiate the vasodilator effects of glyceryl trinitrate and calcium-channel blocks (e.g. nifedipine) and increase the extra-pyramidal side-effects in patients taking neuroleptics (e.g. chlorpromazine).

The risk of liver damage with paracetamol is increased in heavy drinkers, and the risk of dehydration is increased in patients taking diuretics. Chronic use of aspirin and alcohol may increase the potential for gastrointestinal ulceration.

The role of the pharmacist

Drug–nutrient interactions may lead to nutrient deficiencies, reduction in efficacy of drug therapy, or occasionally to toxic reactions. Pharmacists can minimise the potential for such interactions by being aware of:

- Drugs that can influence taste and appetite, and put patients off their food
- Drugs which may cause vitamin and mineral deficiencies; the possibility of prescribing supplements can be discussed with the GP
- Drugs which can cause changes in body weight; if this is a problem the drug may need to be changed
- Interactions between dietary supplements and drugs; incompatible supplements should be avoided
- Interactions between drugs and enteral or parenteral feeds
- The use of meals and snacks as memory joggers to aid drug compliance
- The possible influence of extreme changes in body weight on drug efficacy
- The influence of severe malnutrition on drug dosage
- The need to avoid specific foods and drinks in conjunction with MAOIs
- The need to restrict or avoid alcohol with certain drugs

Further reading

Roe, D. (1989) *Diet and Drug Interactions*. Van Nostrand Reinhold, New York.
Stockley, I. (1991) *Drug Interactions*. Blackwell Scientific Publications, Oxford.

Section 7
Nutritional Support

Chapter 27
The Need for Nutritional Support

Most of us take for granted the ability to eat and drink normally, and we tend to think of malnutrition as a problem only of developing countries. There are people in affluent countries, however, who are at risk of malnutrition because they either cannot eat or cannot absorb the nutrients from a normal diet. Patients with severe burns or those with cancer have increased nutrient requirements and are also at risk of becoming malnourished.

In otherwise healthy, well nourished patients, a temporary reduction in food intake is not too serious. However, in the case of long periods of dietary restriction, some form of nutritional support will be necessary. This is particularly important for children and elderly people because they may have considerably lower reserves of energy and nutrients than healthy adults and are therefore at greater risk of malnutrition.

Malnutrition results in lethargy, poor wound healing, and increased risk of infection and nutritional deficiencies. Severe and long-term food restriction means that the patient will have to draw on existing energy reserves (mainly fat), and some weight loss is inevitable.

Nutritional support is usually taken to mean the provision of specially formulated products in the form of drinks, enteral tube feeds or intravenous infusions. The use of vitamin and mineral preparations is discussed in Chapter 25.

Traditionally, people requiring tube feeds and parenteral nutrition have been kept in hospital, but, as hospital stays become shorter and more people are cared for at home, the need for nutritional support in the community is increasing.

Community pharmacists will be familiar with dispensing prescriptions for enteral feeds and may occasionally encounter patients receiving home parenteral nutrition. Pharmacists therefore need to be aware of these special feeding methods and why people need them, and also to understand some of the problems which both patients and their carers may face.

Who needs nutritional support?

Nutritional support is required by patients who are malnourished or at risk of becoming so. Patients may become malnourished for three basic reasons. These are:

- Inadequate food intake
- Poor absorption of nutrients
- Increased nutrient requirements

Inadequate food intake

Social factors such as poverty or poor kitchen facilities may limit a person's ability to buy and prepare food. Recent bereavement and living alone may result in apathy and depression, resulting in lack of motivation to cook.

Chronic alcoholism is often associated with an inadequate and irregular intake of food not least because drinking alcohol is expensive and financial constraints may mean that priority is given to alcohol instead of food. Heavy drinking also reduces the appetite because energy needs are being met by the alcohol. A bottle of gin provides about 8.4 MJ (2000 kcal) and six pints of beer about 4.3 MJ (1200 kcal).

The possibility of eating disorders should not be forgotten and pharmacists should be aware that individuals buying large quantities of laxatives may be doing so because they have either anorexia or bulimia.

Any condition which leads to pain, e.g. arthritis, may lead to difficulty in both preparing and eating food. Difficulties in swallowing or chewing and the presence of a sore mouth will often limit the variety of food which a person can eat.

Poor appetite or loss of taste may reduce the palatability of food. Drugs such as digoxin, levodopa and lithium can reduce appetite, and taste impairment can be caused by amiodarone, captopril and penicillamine.

Poor absorption

Reduced absorption of nutrients may occur because of intestinal disease such as Crohn's disease, coeliac disease, lactose intolerance, ulcerative colitis and bowel fistulae. Intestinal surgery in which a major part of the small intestine is removed will also lead to failure of nutrient absorption. Any condition which causes vomiting or diarrhoea will lead to poor absorption.

Increased requirements

In conditions such as cancer, the presence of damaged tissue increases energy requirements considerably and even if patients want to eat they may be unable to eat enough to satisfy increased body needs.

Severe burns and major infection may also increase nutritional needs. In fever, which is often caused by infection, each degree Celsius rise in body temperature increases both energy requirements and fluid loss by about 10%. Severe and long-term infection can increase the loss of protein from the body which is likely to lead to muscle wasting unless compensated for by adequate intake.

Recognition of malnutrition

Pharmacists are not used to looking for signs of malnutrition and may be unaware that some of their regular customers are at risk. In hospital a patient's nutritional state is assessed by the use of a dietary history, measurements of height, weight and body fat, clinical examination and laboratory analyses of blood and urine. Even without the facilities for such techniques pharmacists can easily obtain some indication of a patient's nutritional state by asking a few carefully chosen questions.

Questions to ask

- Has the patient noticed weight loss, and, if so, over what period of time?
- What is the patient's normal weight?
- Has recent food intake been any different from usual?
- Have any particular foods been avoided?
- Has appetite been normal?
- Is the patient enjoying food as much as usual?
- Does the patient have any swallowing difficulties or a sore mouth?
- Has the patient suffered from prolonged diarrhoea or vomiting?
- Has the patient suffered any recent illness?
- Does the patient have any condition which causes severe pain?
- Is the patient taking any drugs? If so, which ones?
- Has the patient reduced physical activities because of weakness or fatigue?
- Has there been any change in social circumstances, e.g. bereavement?
- Does the patient feel lethargic, apathetic or depressed?

Physical assessment

Pharmacists who have the facilities should measure body weight and height. From these measurements the body mass index (BMI) can be calculated using the following formula:

$$BMI = \frac{Weight\ in\ kg}{Height\ in\ (m)^2}$$

The normal range for BMI is 20 to 25. A value of under 20 may be indicative of malnutrition.

Weight is not an infallible guide to nutritional state because patients can have a BMI of more than 25 and appear overweight, but still be at risk of malnutrition if they have lost more than 10% of their normal weight in the last month. This is why it is important to ask patients about their normal weight.

Another factor to bear in mind is that the presence of oedema may result in a normal weight measurement in a patient who would be underweight if the excess fluid were to be removed.

Even without the facilities for measuring body weight, pharmacists can still make a great contribution to the detection of malnutrition in the community. An awareness of the reasons for malnutrition, asking the right questions, and making careful observations will all help to assess if a person is at risk of malnutrition.

If malnutrition is suspected, the patient should be referred without delay to the general practitioner. Some form of nutritional support may be necessary. This may be provided via the gastrointestinal tract (enteral nutrition – see Chapter 28) or intravenously (parenteral nutrition – see Chapter 29).

Chapter 28
Enteral Nutrition

Enteral nutrition is taken to mean the provision of energy and nutrients via the gastrointestinal tract. Four categories of enteral nutrition are described:

- Appetising and nourishing foods
- Oral supplements
- Sip feeds
- Tube feeds

These methods of feeding are not mutually exclusive. Some nutrients can be obtained from tube or sip feeding and some from normal foods.

Appetising and nourishing foods

During illness the effort of eating a normal meal can be overwhelming. Patients who are ill may have no appetite for meat and two vegetables, but they will often manage soup, soft rolls, breakfast cereals, sandwiches and desserts made with milk. Milk is a useful source of nutrients so long as lactose intolerance is not a problem.

Fried and fatty foods may be particularly unwelcome and small frequent snacks may be eaten more readily than large meals. Fluid should preferably be high in energy (calories), e.g. milk, fruit juice or glucose drinks.

Problems with eating and drinking may occur for a variety of reasons such as sore mouth and throat, swallowing difficulties and lack of appetite or feeling full too quickly. Specific advice can be given to help alleviate these difficulties.

Sore mouth and throat

- Choose soft moist food
- Offer cold or frozen foods and drinks: they will temporarily numb soreness
- Eat food lukewarm rather than hot
- Avoid acidic fruits such as citrus fruit and tomatoes because they may cause stinging; choose bananas, peaches and pears instead

- Avoid dry foods such as toast, crackers and crispbreads
- Use a mouthwash (e.g. Difflam) or an anaesthetic gel (e.g. Bonjela, Medijel) or spray (e.g. Eludril) just before eating.
- Use an artificial saliva spray (e.g. Glandosane, Luborant or Saliva Orthana) if the mouth is particularly dry
- Administer prescribed analgesics to have the maximum effect at meal-times

Swallowing difficulties

- Eat slowly and chew thoroughly
- Cook food well and avoid chunks of raw or lightly cooked vegetables
- Put fruit and vegetables through a food processor, or mash or sieve them
- Avoid all hard food such as toast and crackers

Feeling full too quickly

- Offer small snacks at short intervals, e.g. every 2–3 hours
- Drink fluid between meals rather than with meals
- Offer a glass of wine or other aperitif; this may stimulate the appetite.

Oral supplements

If the patient is unable to swallow but is not able to eat enough food to maintain adequate nutrition, extra energy (calories) can be provided in the form of oral supplements, which can be mixed with ordinary food, or from commercial drinks which are commonly known as sip feeds.

Soup, milk puddings, yoghurt, ice cream, porridge and milk drinks can be enriched with commercial formulas that contain carbohydrate, fat, protein or a mixture of the three (see Table 28.1). These products can be used in varying proportions and in different recipes to give patients tastes which they like. Supplements in the form of puddings are also available (e.g. Formance, Fortipudding and Maxisorb).

Sip feeds

Sip feeds are liquids which can be used to provide a part or the whole of a patient's required nutritional intake. Most of the products used for sip feeding can also be used as a tube feed; there is a great deal of overlap. Those designed mainly for sip feeding (see Table 28.2) tend to be packed in cartons (sometimes called Tetrabriks) and supplied in assorted flavours. products designed mainly as tube feeds are often packed in glass or plastic bottles and are more frequently unflavoured.

Pharmacists should be able to give advice on the range of flavours available, and patients should not be expected to rely on one product alone.

Individuals may be consuming up to 2 litres a day of these products so monotony can easily be a problem.

Sip feeds can be taken from a glass, cup or feeding beaker or with a straw. Patients should be advised to swallow sip feeds slowly because they may cause diarrhoea if consumed very rapidly. As a rough guide, the contents of one 200 ml glass or carton may be consumed over a period of about 30 minutes. All liquid supplements taste best if they are well chilled but unfortunately there is a greater risk of diarrhoea with cold products.

Tube feeds

If adequate nutrition cannot be achieved by mouth, a liquid feed may be introduced directly into the stomach or intestine via a tube or a surgically inserted catheter.

Who needs tube feeding?

There are four main indications for tube feeding:

- Patients who cannot consume enough food to satisfy nutritional needs because of severe eating and swallowing difficulties. Examples include patients with severe facial injury and cancers of the head, neck and oesophagus, patients with anorexia because of long-standing illness and some cardiac and respiratory disorders.
- Patients with severe intestinal malabsorption including those with Crohn's disease, cystic fibrosis, malignancy or those who have had major gastrointestinal surgery.
- Patients with increased nutritional requirements such as those with major burns, severe injury or cancer.
- Patients with organ failure such as renal or hepatic failure.

Home tube feeding

Tube feeding usually begins in hospital and for some patients continues at home. Home tube feeding allows the patient more freedom and independence and more normal relationships with family and friends. Patients are often happier at home in familiar surroundings and many are able to go back to work either part or full time.

Patient training

Patients should only be allowed to leave hospital once it has been established that they can cope. Tube feeding is an alien concept for most people and the reasons for using it must be carefully explained.

Training will involve care of the equipment and making sure that the

Table 28.1   Oral supplements prescribable under ACBS guidelines (composition/100 ml or 100 g).

Product	Energy kJ (kcal)	CHO g	Fat g	Pr g	Flavour	Pack	Size
General supplements							
Build-Up*,c (Clintec)							
Drink	445 (106)	12.7	3.8	6.2	U, Ch, LL, S, Va	P	38 g
Soup	281 (67)	10.3	1.5	3.6	C, M, Pl	P	38/40 g
Complan*,c (Farley)							
sweet	365 (87)	11.0	2.7	4.0	U, Ch, S	P	58/450 g
savoury	365 (87)	11.0	2.7	4.0	C, M	P	58 g
Formance c (Abbott)	739 (136)	23.9	6.8	4.8	Bu, Ch, Va	Can	142 g
Fortipudding c (Nutricia Clinical)	550 (130)	16	3	10	Ch, Co, Va	Tub	150 g
Maxisorb c (Scientific Hospital Supplies)	565 (135)	9	6	12	Ch, S, Va	P	30 g
Carbohydrate sources							
Caloreen a (Nestlé Clinical)	1674 (400)	96	–	–		P	250 g
Calsip b (Fresenius)	1050 (246)	50	–	–	Ap, Pn, Nu	CT	200 ml
Duobar b (Scientific Hospital Supplies)	2692 (648)	49.9	49.9	–	Nu, S	Bar	45 g
Duocal a (Scientific Hospital Supplies)							
Liquid	628 (150)	23.4	7.1	–		B	250 ml
MCT	2042 (486)	74	23.2	–		P	400 g
Super-soluble	1988 (470)	72.7	22.3	–		P	400 g
Fortical a (Cow & Gate Nutricia)	1050 (246)	62.0	–	–	U, Ap, Apr, Bl, L, Or	B	200 ml
Hycal a (SmithKline Beecham)	1035 (243)	49.5	–	–	Bl, L, Or, Rs	B	171 ml
Maxijul a (Scientific Hospital Supplies)							
Liquid	800 (187)	50	–	–	U, Bl, LL,	CT	200 ml
Super-soluble	1500 (360)	95	–	–	Or	P	140 g, 200 g, 2.5 kg
Maxijul LE a (Scientific Hospital Supplies)	1500 (360)	96	–	–		P	100 g/2 kg
Polycal b (Nutricia Clinical)							
Liquid	1050 (246)	61.5	–	–	Ap, Bl, L, Nu, Or	CT	200 ml
Powder	1610 (380)	94.5	–	–		P	400 g
Polycose a (Abbott)	1610 (380)	94.0	–	–		P	350 g
Vitajoule b (Vitaflo)	1610 (380)	96.0	–	–		P	125 g/200 g/500 g / 2.5 kg/25 kg

Cont.

Table 28.1   Cont.

Product	Energy kJ (kcal)	CHO g	Fat g	Pr g	Flavour	Pack	Size
Fat sources							
Alembicol D[a] (Alembicol Products)	3738 (890)	–	99	–		B	4 kg
Calogen[a] (Scientific Hospital Supplies)	1850 (450)	–	50	–	–	B	250 ml/1L
Liquigen[a] (Scientific Hospital Supplies)	1700 (400)	–	52	–	–	B	250 ml/1 L
MCT Oil[a]	3738 (890)	–	99	–	–	B	250/950 ml/1 L
Protein sources							
Casilan[b] (Heinz)	1600 (376)	<0.5	1.8	90.0	U	P	250 g
Maxipro Super Soluble[c] (Scientific Hospital Supplies)	1662 (393)	<5.0	6.0	80.0	U	P	200 g/1 kg
Pro-Mod[a] (Abbott)	1788 (426)	10.2	9.1	75.8	U	P	275 g

* Not prescribable

Note: All products gluten-free.

[a] Lactose-free; [b] Traces of lactose; [c] Contains lactose.

Abbreviations: CHO = carbohydrate; Pr = protein

Key to flavours: Ap, apple; Apr, apricot; As, asparagus; B, banana; Bl, blackcurrant; C, chicken; Ca, caramel; Ch, chocolate; CM, chocolate mint; Co, coffee; DB, dandelion and burdock; Eg, eggnog; FF, fruits of the forest; FP, fruit punch; G, grapefruit; L, lemon; LL, lemon and lime; M, mushroom; Mc, mocha; Mn, mandarin; Nu, nut; Or, orange; P, peach; P&Or, peach and orange; Pl, potato and leek; Pn, pineapple; Rs, raspberry; S, strawberry; TF, tropical fruit; Veg, vegetable; U, unflavoured; Va, vanilla.

Key to packs: B, bottle; CT, carton; P, powder; TB, tetrabrik.

Table 28.2 Products used as sip feeds.

Advera (Abbott)	Fortifresh (Nutricia Clinical)
Calsip (Fresenius)	Fortijuice (Nutricia Clinical)
Complan (Crookes)	Fortimel (Nutricia Clinical)
Enlive (Abbott)	Fortisip (Nutricia Clinical)
Enrich (Abbott)	Fresubin (Fresenius)
Ensure (Abbott)	Protein Forte (Fresenius)
Ensure Plus (Abbott)	Provide (Fresenius)

Note: For flavours, pack sizes and nutritional composition, see Tables 28.1 and 28.4.

patient can place the feeding tube correctly in the gastrointestinal tract. Correct storage of feeds and ordering and delivery procedures should also be explained.

What is also important is that the patient can recognise complications that may occur and know how to deal with emergencies until help arrives. Arrangements should be made for liaison with the nutrition support team in the local hospital, the general practitioner, the district nurse and the community pharmacist. The patient must be clear about where to go for help and supplies of feeds and equipment.

Choice of feed

A large number of tube feeds are available, and it is important that community pharmacists understand the basic differences between them. One feed cannot necessarily be substituted for another. The most recent British National Formulary or Drug Tariff should be consulted for prescribable indications.

The choice of feed is the responsibility of a dietitian and depends on the patient's nutritional requirements. Other related factors taken into account include particular characteristics of the feed such as energy density, non-protein energy : nitrogen ratio and osmolality, and the patient's capacity for digestion and absorption, including specific intolerances to lactose, gluten or milk protein.

Energy density

Most patients can be fed successfully using products with an energy density of 420 kJ (100 kcal)/100 ml (1 kcal/ml), but occasionally a patient may not be able to tolerate the volume of fluid necessary to provide the required amount of energy. Most patients require about 8.4 MJ (2000 kcal)day and this is equivalent to 2 litres of a feed which provides 1 kcal/ml. If this amount of fluid cannot be tolerated, a product containing 630 kJ (150 kcal/100 ml (1.5 kcal/ml) may be used instead. These include Ensure Plus (Abbott and Fresubin 750 MCT.

Non-protein energy : nitrogen ratio

This is defined as the ratio of energy derived from non-protein sources (i.e. carbohydrate and fat) in the feed to the amount of nitrogen and is expressed in kcal/g of nitrogen. Patients in different catabolic states need different ratios (see Table 28.3).

Table 28.3 Approximate guide to non-protein energy : nitrogen ratios for different patients.

Burns patients	100:1
Catabolic patients	120:1
Non-catabolic patients	200:1

Osmolality

Osmolality is defined as the molar concentration of solute in a solution and is expressed in terms of mosmol/kg solvent.

A feed with a high osmolality (> 500 mosmol/kg) is likely to draw fluid into the gut and cause osmotic diarrhoea. Feeds which are isotonic with plasma are tolerated best and have an osmalality of 280–300 mosmol/kg. Most standard feeds fall into this category.

If a feed with high osmolality is used, diarrhoea can be prevented by introducing the feed slowly. Dilution of the feed is not considered necessary.

Capacity for digestion and absorption

Some patients have a reduced ability to break down and absorb nutrients (e.g. patients with pancreatic insufficiency or severe malabsorption syndromes). They may be prescribed a feed in which the protein is pre-digested (an elemental feed – see below), rather than one which contains whole protein.

Lactose intolerance may be a problem in some patients and a lactose-free feed is usually chosen. Some feeds are low in lactose (< 0.1 g/100 ml), providing less than 2 g of lactose per day, and these are also likely to be tolerated by the majority of patients. Some patients are intolerant to gluten but most feeds are gluten-free.

Types of feeds

There are two main types of tube feeds, standard (whole protein) and elemental.

Standard feeds

Standard feeds (see Table 28.4) are generally suitable and cost-effective for most tube-fed patients and tend to be used wherever possible. They contain

Table 28.4 Standard (whole protein) enteral feeds prescribable under ACBS guidelines (composition/100 ml).

Product	Energy kJ (kcal)	CHO g	Fat g	Pr g	Flavour	Pack	Size
Advera[b] (Abbott)	532 (126)	20.3	2.2	5.9	Ch, Or	Can	237 ml
Clinifeed Iso[a] (Nestlé)	420 (100)	13.1	4.1	2.8	Va	Can	375 ml
Clinutren[b] (Nestlé Clinical)							
Iso	420 (100)	14.0	3.3	3.8	Ch, Co, S, Rs, Va	Pot	200 ml
1.5	630 (150)	21.0	5.0	5.5	Apr, B, Ch, Rs, S, Va	Pot	200 ml
Enlive[b] (Abbott)	530 (125)	27.2	4.0	–	Ap, FP, G, LL, Or, P, Pn, S	CT	200 ml
Enrich[b,c] (Abbott)	436 (104)	15.3	3.5	3.8	Ch, Va	Can	250 ml
Ensure[b] (Abbott)							
sweet	420 (100)	13.7	3.5	3.5	Bl, Ch, Co, Eg, Nu, Va	B/Can	237/250/946 ml
savoury	420 (100)	13.4	3.4	4.2	As, C, M	Can	250 ml
Ensure Plus[b] (Abbott)	630 (150)	20.0	5.0	6.3	Va	B	200/500 ml/1 L
Entera[b] (Fresenius)	630 (150)	18.8	5.8	5.6	B, Bl, Bu, CM, Or, Pn, S, Va, Veg, Nu	CT	200 ml
Fortifresh[b] (Nutricia Clinical)	654 (155)	21.1	5.0	6.5	Bl, Mn, Rs	CT	200 ml
Fortijuice[b] (Nutricia Clinical)	523 (125)	28.4	–	4.0	Apr, Bl, DB, LL	CT	200 ml
Fortimel[a] (Nutricia Clinical)	420 (100)	10.4	2.1	9.7	S, FF, Va	CT	200 ml
Fortisip[d] (Nutricia Clinical)	630 (150)	17.9	6.5	5	B, Ch, Mu, Or, S, TF, U	B	200 ml
Frebini[b] (Fresenius)	420 (100)	13.5	4.0	2.5	U	B	200 ml
Fresubin (Fresenius)							
Fresubin liquid[d]	420 (100)	13.8	3.4	3.8	Bl, Ch, Mc, Nu, P, Va	CT/B	200/500 ml
Fresubin Isofibre[c,d]	420 (100)	13.8	3.4	3.8	U	B/Bag	500 ml
Fresubin 750 MCT[1,d]	630 (150)	17	6	7.5	Va	B	500 ml
Jevity[b,c] (Abbott)	420 (100)	13.4	3.5	4.2	U	B	500 ml/1 L/1.5 L
Jevity Plus[b,c] (Abbott)	504 (120)	16.1	–	5.6	U	B	1 L/1.5 L
Nutrini[b] (Nutricia Clinical)							
Nutrini Extra	630 (150)	18.8	6.8	3.4	U	B/Bag	200 ml/500 ml
Nutrini Standard	420 (100)	12.2	4.5	2.8	U	B/Bag	200 ml/500 ml

Cont.

Table 28.4 Cont.

Product	Energy kJ (kcal)	CHO g	Fat g	Pr g	Flavour	Pack	Size
Nutrison (Nutricia Clinical)							
Nutrison Energy[1,d]	630 (150)	18.4	5.8	6	U	B	500 ml/1 L
Nutrison Fibre[c,d]	420 (100)	12.3	3.9	4	U	B	500 ml/1 L
Nutrison Standard[d]	420 (100)	12.3	3.9	4	U	B	500 ml/1 L
Osmolite[b] (Abbott)	420 (100)	13.4	3.5	4.2	U	Can/B	250/500 ml
Paediasure (Abbott)							
Liquid[2,b]	420 (100)	11.2	5.0	2.8	Va	Can	250 ml
Liquid with fibre[c]	421 (100)	11.2	5.0	2.8	Va	Can	250 ml
Perative[1,b] (Abbott)	551 (130)	17.7	3.7	6.6	U	Can/B	237 ml/1 L
Protein Forte[1,a] (Fresenius)	420 (100)	9.5	2.6	10	Ch, S, Va	TB	200 mL
Provide[1,b] (Fresenius)	525 (125)	7.5	<1	3.7	Ap, Bl, Ch, CC, LL, Ml, Or, P	CT	200 ml
Sondalis (Nestlé Clinical)							
Fibre[b,c]	420 (100)	12.5	3.9	3.8	U	B	500 ml/1 L
ISO[b]	420 (100)	12.5	3.9	3.8	U	B	500 ml/1 L
1.5[b]	420 (100)	12.5	3.9	3.8	U	B	500 ml/1 L
Survimed OPD[b] (Fresenius)	420 (100)	15.0	2.6	4.5	U	B/Bag	500 ml
Triosorbon[a] (Merck)	420 (100)	11.9	4.0	4.0	U	P	85 g

Note: All products gluten-free except Fresubin Plus F (muesli).
[1] Prescribable in the community as a nutritional supplement only.
[2] For children (not prescribable for infants under 1 year).
[a] Contains lactose; [b] Lactose-free; [c] Contains added dietary fibre; [d] Practically lactose-free (0.1 g/100 ml).

Abbreviation: CHO = carbohydrate
For key to flavours and packs see Table 28.1

undigested protein in the form of skimmed milk, soya protein, whey protein or caseinates. Most contain some milk protein.

Fat is in the form of triglycerides, some of which contain long chain fatty acids and some of which contain medium chain fatty acids. Medium chain triglycerides are more easily digested than long chain triglycerides. Various oils such as peanut oil, coconut oil and corn oil are used as a source of fat.

Carbohydrate is provided in the form of glucose, glucose polymers (e.g. maltodextrins), sucrose and hydrolysed maize (corn) starch. A few standard feeds contain non-starch polysaccharides (dietary fibre). These include Enrich, Jevity (Abbott) and Nutrison Fibre (Nutricia Clinical).

Most, but not all, standard tube feeds are both lactose-free and gluten-free.

Elemental feeds

Elemental feeds (see Table 28.5) provide protein, carbohydrate and fat in a more easily digested form than standard tube feeds and are therefore also known as predigested feeds.

Instead of whole protein they contain amino acids, peptides or hydrolysed protein. Most of the fat is in the form of medium chain triglycerides, and carbohydrate is provided by glucose and other simple carbohydrates.

Elemental feeds are more expensive than standard feeds and usually more unpalatable because they contain less fat. They also tend to have a higher osmolality which means that they must be introduced slowly into the feeding tube.

For these reasons, elemental feeds tend to be restricted to use in severe digestive disorders such as pancreatic disease or in conditions of severe malabsorption including short bowel syndrome, bowel fistulas and acute Crohn's disease.

All elemental feeds are gluten-free, milk-protein free and either lactose-free or low in lactose.

Routes of administration

Enteral feeds can be administered by nasogastric or nasoduodenal tube or via an oesophagostomy, gastrostomy, duodenostomy or jejunostomy catheter (Fig. 28.1). The most commonly used route for short-term enteral feeding is the nasogastric tube. Nasal passage of a tube avoids the need for surgery. If disease of the upper gastrointestinal tract makes the passage of a tube difficult, then it can be done under local anaesthesia.

Enterostomy catheters must be put in place by surgery and tend to be used where enteral feeding is used for longer than six months.

Enteral feeding equipment

The equipment used for enteral feeding consists of nasogastric feeding tubes or enterostomy catheters, feeding bottles, administration sets and delivery pumps (Fig. 28.2).

Table 28.5 Elemental feeds prescribable under ACBS guidelines (composition/100 ml).

Product	Energy kJ (kcal)	CHO g	Fat g	Pr g	Flavour	Pack	Size
Elemental 028[1],[a] (Scientific Hospital Supplies)							
028 powder	323 (76)	14.1	1.3	2.0	U, Or	P	100 g
028 extra powder	358 (85)	11.0	3.5	2.5	U, Or	P	100 g
028 extra liquid	358 (85)	11.0	3.5	2.5	U, Or	P	100 g
Emsogen[1],[a] (Scientific Hospital Supplies)	358 (85)	11.0	3.5	2.5	U, Or	P	100 g
Nutrison Pepti[1],[a] (Nutricia Clinical)							
Liquid	420 (100)	18.8	1.0	4.0	U	B, CP	500 ml/1 L
Powder	415 (98)	18.6	1.0	3.6	U	P	126 g
Peptamen[a] (Clintec)	420 (100)	12.7	3.9	4	U, Or, S, Va	Can/B	250/500 ml

Note: All products gluten-free.
[1] Flavoured varieties have slightly different nutrient content.
[a] Lactose-free.

key to flavours: Or, orange; S, strawberry; U, unflavoured; Va, vanilla.
Key to packs: B, bottle; CP, collapsible pack; P, powder.

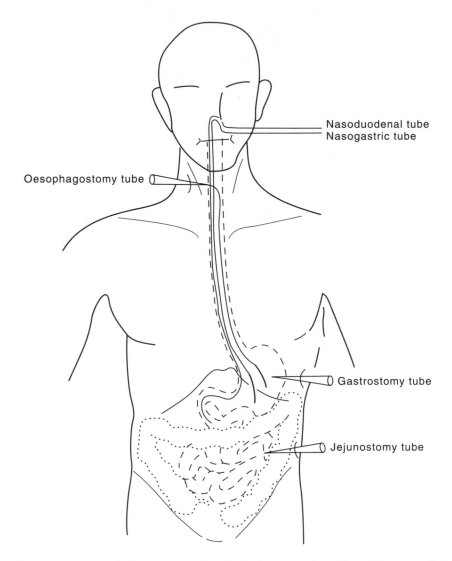

Fig. 28.1   Routes of administration for tube feeds. (Reproduced from *The Manual of Dietetics*, Thomas, B. (ed.) 1988, with kind permission of Blackwell Scientific Publications, Oxford.)

Methods of administration

Feeds can be given by bolus or by continuous administration, but for patients being fed at home a common procedure is to give the feed continuously for 10–12 hours during the night and then disconnect it during the day. This allows the patient freedom from the administration set during the day when they can sometimes take food by mouth and participate in family meals.

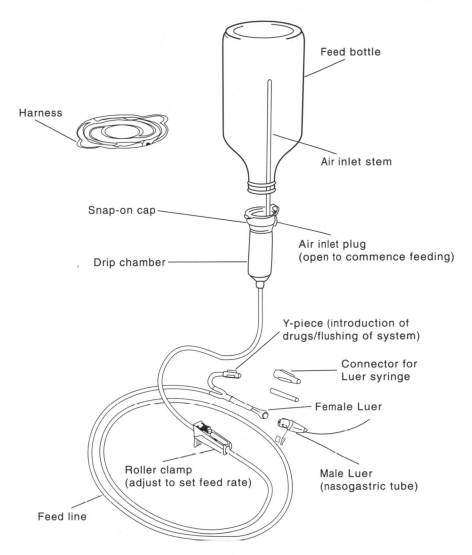

Fig. 28.2   A nasogastric feeding set. (Reproduced with kind permission of Fresenius.)

Complications

Complications associated with tube feeding are common but rarely life threatening. Nevertheless, they can cause the patient a great deal of suffering, and may lead to inadequate energy and nutrient intake.

Gastrointestinal disturbances

One of the commonest complications of tube feeding is diarrhoea. This may be caused by too rapid introduction of large volumes of feed, particularly if the feed has a high osmolality. Bacterial contamination of the feed, lactose intolerance or the administration of antibiotics can all lead to diarrhoea in tube-fed patients. Cold feeds can also cause problems so unopened feeds should not be stored in the refrigerator.

Constipation is likely to be a problem during tube feeding but patients may often just need the reassurance that a once-weekly bowel movement is quite normal in their circumstances. A few feeds containing dietary fibre are now available (see Table 28.4) and may be useful for improving gut function.

Mechanical problems

Mechanical problems may arise as a result of tube insertion. These include regurgitation, aspiration and oesophagitis. Regurgitation of feeds is often a problem in patients who are being fed overnight; it can be prevented by raising the head of the bed by about 30°.

Some patients inadvertently remove the tube, and tubes can become blocked. Blockage can occur as a result of drug administration (see p.281).

Metabolic problems

Water and electrolyte disturbances seem to be the most common metabolic problems associated with tube feeding. Fluid intake and output should be checked regularly and serum electrolytes monitored frequently.

Even though nutritionally complete feeds contain vitamins and minerals, there is still a risk of deficiencies especially where gastrointestinal losses are excessive. Patients should be monitored regularly and additional vitamins and minerals given if necessary.

Psychological problems

For tube feeding to be a success, patients need time to accept it, and they need a great deal of encouragement. It can be difficult to adjust to the presence of tubes, and sleep disturbance may be a problem for patients being fed at night. It is not surprising that depression is a common problem.

Food deprivation is an unnatural state and this can be minimised by encouraging the patient to eat some normal food. Participation in family mealtimes should be encouraged wherever possible.

Contamination

Enteral feeds and equipment can easily become contaminated, and while strict asepsis is not necessary, rigorous hygienic procedures should be followed. Patients may be tube fed at home for prolonged periods, and with time they may become more casual in the preparation of feeds and handling of equipment.

Pharmacists should remind patients of the need to adhere to the following procedures:

- All equipment should be kept in sealed packages until ready for use.
- The sink, taps and work surfaces should be cleaned and then disinfected before handling the feed; care must be taken in making up the disinfectant (e.g. Milton) to the required strength.
- The enteral feed should not be handled in close proximity to other food.
- Disposable gloves should be used to handle feeds and equipment or the hands should be washed and thoroughly disinfected.
- If feeds have to be transferred to another container, the outsides of the containers and any bottle or can openers should be disinfected immediately before use.
- The feed should be administered immediately after preparing the administration set.
- Unused feeds in opened containers should be kept covered on the top shelf of a refrigerator for no more than 24 hours and then discarded.
- Opened feeds should not be stored underneath products such as raw or thawing meat because of the risk of blood dropping on to the feed container.
- Disposable equipment should never be reused.
- Sip feeds should be handled with equally careful attention and should never be left opened at the side of the patient's bed for longer than 4 hours.
- Feeds should not be used after their 'use before' date.
- All feeds should be examined carefully for any signs of thickening, lumps or separation.
- Sterile feeds should never be left hanging for more than 24 hours at a time.
- Non-sterile feeds, including powdered feeds may up with water, should never be left hanging for more than 4 hours.
- The feeding tube should be flushed with tap water at least once every 24 hours (use sterile water if the patient is particularly susceptible to infection).

Monitoring

Complete nutritional assessment of the patient will be carried out at the start of feeding in hospital and the patient will need to return to the hospital regularly for monitoring of plasma electrolytes, urea and glucose. Initially this is likely to be every week and then monthly.

Once at home the patient should be weighed at least weekly, if not more often, and the daily energy intake calculated from the amount of feed consumed. Some patients may also be asked to record fluid intake and output.

Drugs

Patients being tube fed may need drugs and there may be incompatibilities. Specific interactions between drugs and enteral feeds are considered in

Chapter 26, but the following general principles should be considered when administering any drug to a tube fed patient.

- Review the need for all drugs continually: is the drug really necessary?
- Consider the possibility of drug–nutrient interactions in enteral feeds, e.g. antacids, anticoagulants, phenytoin and theophylline (see Chapter 26).
- Aim, if practicable, to leave a gap of 2 hours between the administration of a feed and a drug.
- Use aqueous solutions of drugs wherever possible rather than elixirs, emulsions, suspensions, pulverised tablets or powders emptied from capsules.
- Never put drugs into the feeding bottle.
- Always stop the feed and wash out the tube with water before and after giving the drug.
- Remember that antibiotics are associated with diarrhoea in tube-fed patients.
- Consider other routes of administration, e.g. rectal, intramuscular or intravenous.

The role of the pharmacist

Enteral feeding in hospital is managed by a nutritional support team which includes a pharmacists, a dietitian and a nutrition nurse. Patients receiving nutritional support at home are not under such constant and specialised supervision and rely to a great extent on the support of their family and the primary health care team which includes community pharmacists.

Pharmacists can make the following contributions to the successful management of enteral feeding in the community:

- Offer appropriate dietary advice in cases of specific feeding difficulties such as painful mouth, swallowing difficulties and poor appetite.
- Provide information of flavours and convenient packs for patients using oral supplements and sip feeds.
- Remind patients of the need to adhere to strict procedures of hygiene when handling enteral feeds and equipment.
- Recognise the complications of tube feeding and ensure that there is no delay in seeking specialised help where necessary.
- Supply feeds.

Further reading

BAPEN (1994) *Enteral and Parenteral Nutrition in the Community*. British Association for Parenteral and Enteral Nutrition, Maidenhead, Berkshire.

BAPEN (1998) *Ethical and Legal Aspects of Clinical Hydration and Nutritional Support*. British Association for Parenteral and Enteral Nutrition. Maidenhead, Berkshire.

BAPEN (1999) *Current Perspectives on Enteral Nutrition in Adults.* British Association for Parenteral and Enteral Nutrition, Maidenhead Berkshire.

Grant, A. & Todd, E. (1987) *Enteral and Parenteral Nutrition*, Blackwell Scientific Publications, Oxford.

King's Fund Centre (1992) A Positive Approach to Nutrition as Treatment. Report of a working party on the role of enteral and parenteral feeding in hospital and at home. The King's Fund Centre, London.

Chapter 29
Parenteral Nutrition

Parenteral nutrition is the aseptic delivery of nutrients directly into the circulatory system. This route may be used as the sole source of nutrition, in which case it is known as total parenteral nutrition (TPN), although most patients do manage to take some food by mouth.

Who needs it?

The indications for parenteral nutrition are basically the same as those for tube feeding. In deciding which of the two methods to use, the most important factor to take into account is gut function. Parenteral nutrition is a highly specialised technique, not without hazards, and should be reserved for those patients whose guts are not functioning.

Some specific conditions in which parenteral feeding is common required include:

- Crohn's disease
- Radiation enteritis
- Thrombosis of the mesenteric artery or vein
- Short bowel syndrome
- Bowel fistulae
- Acute pancreatitis
- Malignancy of the intestine
- Extensive bowel resection.

Home parenteral nutrition (HPN)

Home parenteral nutrition (HPN) was first practised in the UK in 1977. Developments in the techniques of intravenous feeding now allow patients to be maintained for many years, if not indefinitely, without the need to eat. When patients require parenteral nutrition for more than about a month, it is often possible to allow them to continue at home.

Patient training

The administration of HPN requires meticulous attention to detail, and successful training may take 3–4 weeks to complete. Patients should only be allowed home once they are able to demonstrate competence in handling the equipment.

In all aspects of patient training the support of the rest of the family or household is essential. Both the patient and another member of the family are usually trained in all the techniques. One of the most important factors to be explained to the patient is the need for strict aseptic technique in manipulation of the intravenous catheter and feeding lines.

Home facilities

A large refrigerator will be required for storing the bags of infusion solutions. Extra shelves are needed for storing all the accessories required for administration. Drip stands should move easily over domestic carpets. If possible, the patient should have two drip stands, one for upstairs and one for downstairs.

An aseptically clean work surface is required for the preparation of equipment and dressings. A telephone is usually considered essential for contacting the hospital or community health care workers in case of emergencies.

Composition of the feeds

Intravenous feeds provide energy and fluid and also contain amino acids, electrolytes, vitamins, minerals and trace elements.

Energy

The energy requirements of most patients can be met on a regimen of about 8.4 MJ (2000 kcal)/day. Glucose can be used as the sole energy source but, if large amounts of glucose (> 300 g/day) are given intravenously, there is a risk of hyperglycaemia and insulin may be necessary. Fat does not cause hyperglycaemia and some of the energy is usually provided by fat. Fat is also required as a source of the essential fatty acids.

Fluid

For most patients a normal urine output is obtained with infusions of 2 litres of solutions daily. Fluid requirements can increase quite considerably if the patient has a fever.

Amino acids

Protein is provided in the form of amino acids. All the essential amino acids are included, together with a wide variety of non-essential amino acids. This is because the synthesis of all amino acids, both essential and non-essential, may be impaired in patients who are ill.

Electrolytes

The need for electrolytes such as potassium and sodium varies considerably from patient to patient, and also during any one patient's course of parenteral nutrition. Potassium requirements, for example, may be high at first because of reversal of tissue breakdown. Patients should be monitored regularly and the parenteral prescription changed as necessary.

Minerals and trace elements

Requirements for minerals and trace elements are less than on a normal diet, because such a small proportion of the dietary intake is absorbed from the small intestine.

It is unlikely that patients on short-term intravenous feeding will be deficient in trace elements, but deficiencies are often a problem in patients fed long term. If not added to the infusion bag, zinc is usually the first trace element to become deficient, but deficiencies of chromium copper, molybdenum and selenium may also occur after several weeks or months.

Vitamins

Vitamins are required in at least the same amounts as in the normal diet. If a patient has anaemia, extra vitamin B_{12} and folic acid may be required, and additional vitamin C may be needed by patients after surgery.

Vitamin preparations are extremely unstable in infusion fluids. Vitamin A is susceptible to light, and vitamin C is prone to oxidation. Vitamins must therefore be added separately as well as aseptically to the infusion fluids and used as soon as possible, preferably within 24 hours and certainly within 7 days.

This presents HPN patients with a problem. Vitamins are normally added in a hospital sterile production unit and patients who live near to a hospital may be able to collect their pre-prepared bags at regular intervals. Some companies also provide pre-prepared bags. Alternatively, patients may be trained to make aseptic additions of vitamins in their own infusion fluids. Another option is to give vitamins separately as a once a week intramuscular injection, or even as an oral supplement if the patient is able to absorb them.

Preparation of the feed

Intravenous feeds are prepared under strict aseptic conditions. The feeds are usually made up from commercially available mixtures of amino acids (e.g. Aminoplasmal, Aminoplex, FreAmine, Synthamin and Vamin), glucose, fat (e.g. Intralipid) and electrolytes. Solutions of vitamins (e.g. Multibionta, Solivito N and Vitlipid N) and trace elements (e.g. Addamel and Additrace) may be added separately. One day's feed is usually supplied in a 3-litre plastic bag.

It is also possible to buy ready-prepared bags with a shelf life of 90 days which only require the addition of lipid and vitamins. These are particularly useful for HPN patients.

Route of administration

The normal route of administration for long-term intravenous feeding is through a large central vein. This is because most intravenous feeds are hypertonic and would cause thrombosis if infused into a peripheral vein. The larger volume of blood in central veins allows for rapid dilution of the infusion, and the potential for damage to the vein is much less.

The catheter is inserted under local anaesthesia in strict aseptic conditions. The catheter tip lies in the superior vena cava and the proximal end is tunnelled under the skin to emerge at the front of the chest. The catheter is anchored to a Dacron cuff which lies in the skin tunnel.

Only nutrients should be infused through the catheter. It is very important to remember that drugs should never be introduced via the feeding catheter.

Equipment

The basic equipment for intravenous feeding includes the catheter, a pump and a drip stand. A typical home administration set if shown in Fig. 29.1

The surgically inserted catheter is attached via a giving set to the pump which controls the rate of administration of the infusion. During the time when the patient is not attached to the feed, the giving set can be removed and the catheter flushed with saline to maintain its patency. The catheter is then covered with a sterile dressing which enables the patient to go to work or otherwise maintain a normal life.

Complications of parenteral nutrition

Parenteral nutrition is not without hazards. These include infections, metabolic complications and mechanical problems. Psychological and social problems are similar to those described in association with tube feeding (see p. 269), but may be more extreme because the patient is able to take much less by mouth.

Infections

If the catheter and giving set are not maintained under strict aseptic conditions, it is likely that infection will result. Infection at the exit site will manifest itself as pain, redness and swelling, and patients with these symptoms should inform the hospital at once and stop using the catheter. Patients should also be referred to hospital urgently if they have symptoms of fever;

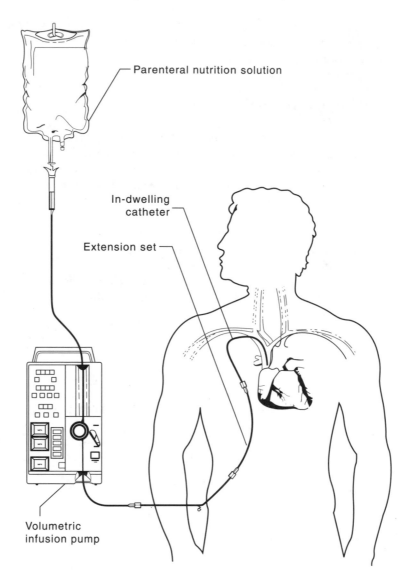

Parenteral nutrition solution

In-dwelling
catheter

Extension set

Volumetric
infusion pump

Fig. 29.1 Home parenteral nutrition administration set. (Reproduced with kind permission of Caremark Ltd.)

such symptoms may be caused by septicaemia. The catheter may need to be removed and antibacterial therapy given.

Metabolic complications

Metabolic complications include water and electrolyte imbalances, trace element deficiencies, hyperglycaemia and hypoglycaemia. Most of these problems can be overcome by careful monitoring of blood levels.

The risk of hyperglycaemia is reduced if the feed is administered slowly and if fat is used to meet some of the energy requirements. Patients with severe glucose intolerance will need insulin.

Hypoglycaemia may be caused by abrupt cessation of the infusion. If this is a problem, the patient should be taught to reduce the flow rate gradually towards the end of a feed.

Mechanical problems

Pneumothorax and air embolism are possible complications of the catheterisation procedure, but are not usually problematical once the patient has been stabilised on the intravenous feed.

One problem to be aware of is a blocked catheter. If this happens, the flow of nutrient solution will cease and a blood clot will form at the catheter tip. Blockage of catheters can best be prevented by ensuring an adequate flow of infusion fluid at all times – probably with a pump. Empty fluid containers should be changed, immediately, and giving lines should never be allowed to become kinked. When the giving set is changed the time between disconnection of the old set and the connection of the new set should be kept to a minimum.

Monitoring of HPN patients

All patients receiving parenteral nutrition will be monitored regularly in hospital and should not be allowed home until they are stabilised on the regimen. Patients are reviewed shortly after discharge and then subsequently at 1- to 2-month intervals.

Routine investigations include the measurement of blood levels of electrolytes, urea and albumin. Fluid balance will also be checked and some patients may be trained to measure fluid input and urine output at home. In patients who need prolonged parenteral nutrition, blood samples are analysed for trace elements and vitamins. Adjustments are made to the nutrient regimen if necessary.

One of the most important things to remember about HPN is that it is usually used for prolonged periods. Because patients in hospital are usually fed for relatively short periods, complications such as trace element deficiencies do not have time to develop. Patients on HPN should have regular biochemical monitoring.

Further reading (see also Chapter 28)

Lee, H.A. & Venkat Raman, G. (1990) *A Handbook of Parenteral Nutrition. Hospital and Home Applications.* Chapman & Hall, London.

Appendix 1
Dietary Reference Values

Estimated Average Requirements (EAR) for energy

Age	Males	Females
	EAR MJ/d (kcal/d)	
0–3 months	2.28 (545)	2.16 (515)
4–6 months	2.89 (690)	2.69 (645)
7–9 months	3.44 (825)	3.20 (765)
10–12 months	3.85 (920)	3.61 (865)
1–3 years	5.15 (1230)	4.86 (1165)
4–6 years	7.16 (1715)	6.46 (1545)
7–10 years	8.24 (1970)	7.28 (1740)
11–14 years	9.27 (2220)	7.92 (1845)
15–18 years	11.51 (2755)	8.83 (2110)
19–50 years	10.60 (2550)	8.10 (1940)
51–59 years	10.60 (2550)	8.00 (1900)
60–64 years	9.93 (2380)	7.99 (1900)
65–74 tears	9.71 (2330)	7.96 (1900)
75 + years	8.77 (2100)	7.61 (1810)
Pregnancy		+0.80[1] (200)
Lactation		
1 month		+1.90 (450)
2 months		+2.20 (530)
3 months		+2.40 (570)
4–6 months (Group 1)[2]		+2.00 (480)
4–6 months (Group 2)		+2.40 (570)
>6 months (Group 1)		+1.00 (240)
>6 months (Group 2)		+2.30 (550)

[1] last trimester only.
[2] Mothers not wholly breast feeding.
Crown copyright. Reproduced with the permission of the Controller of The Stationery Office.

Dietary Reference Values for fat and carbohydrate for adults as a percentage of daily total energy intake (percentage of food energy)

	Individual minimum	Population average	Individual maximum
Saturated fatty acids		10 (11)	
Cis-polyunsaturated fatty acids		6 (6.5)	10
	n-3 0.2		
	n-6 1.0		
Cis-monosaturated fatty acids		12 (13)	
Trans fatty acids		2 (2)	
Total fatty acids		30 (32.5)	
Total fat		33 (35)	
Non-milk extrinsic sugars	0	10 (11)	
Intrinsic and milk sugars and starch		37 (39)	
Total carbohydrate		47 (50)	
Non-starch polysaccharide (g/d)	12	18	24

The average percentage contribution to total energy does not total 100% because figures for protein and alcohol are excluded. Protein intakes average 15% of total energy which is above the RNI. It is recognised that many individuals will derive some energy from alcohol, and this has been assumed to average 5% approximating to current intakes. However, some groups might not drink alcohol, and for some purposes nutrient intakes as a proportion of food energy (without alcohol) might be useful. Therefore average figures are given as percentages both of total energy and, in parenthesis, of food energy.

Reference Nutrient Intakes for protein

Age	Reference Nutrient Intakes g/d
0–3 months	12.5
4–6 months	12.7
7–9 months	13.7
10–12 months	14.9
1–3 years	14.5
4–6 years	19.7
7–10 years	28.3
Males:	
11–14 years	42.1
15–18 years	55.2
19–50 years	55.5
50 + years	53.3
Females:	
11–14 years	41.2
15–18 years	45.0
19–50 years	45.0
50 + years	46.5
Pregnancy[1]	+ 6
Lactation[1]	
0–4 months	+ 11
4 + months	+ 8

[1] To be added to adult requirement through all stages of pregnancy and lactation. Crown copyright. Reproduced with the permission of the Controller of The Stationery Office.

Reference Nutrient Intakes for vitamins

Age	Thiamin mg/d	Riboflavin mg/d	Niacin (nicotinic acid equivalent) mg/d	Vitamin B$_6$ mg/d[1]	Vitamin B$_{12}$ µg/d	Folate µg/d	Vitamin C mg/d	Vitamin A µg/d	Vitamin D µg/d
0–3 months	0.2	0.4	3	0.2	0.3	50	25	350	8.5
4–6 months	0.2	0.4	3	0.2	0.3	50	25	350	8.5
7–9 months	0.2	0.4	4	0.3	0.4	50	25	350	7
10–12 months	0.3	0.4	5	0.4	0.4	50	25	350	7
1–3 years	0.5	0.6	8	0.7	0.5	70	30	400	7
4–6 years	0.7	0.8	11	0.9	0.8	100	30	500	–
7–10 years	0.7	1.0	12	1.0	1.0	150	30	500	–
Males									
11–14 years	0.9	1.2	15	1.2	1.2	200	35	600	–
15–18 years	1.1	1.3	18	1.5	1.5	200	40	700	–
19–50 years	1.0	1.3	17	1.4	1.5	200	40	700	–
50 + years	0.9	1.3	16	1.4	1.5	200	40	700	**
Females									
11–14 years	0.7	1.1	12	1.0	1.2	200	35	600	–
15–18 years	0.8	1.1	14	1.2	1.5	200	40	600	–
19–50 years	0.8	1.1	13	1.2	1.5	200	40	600	–
50 + years	0.8	1.1	12	1.2	1.5	200	40	600	**
Pregnancy	+ 0.1***	+ 0.3	*	*	*	+ 100	+ 10	+ 100	10
Lactation:									
0–4 months	+ 0.2	+ 0.5	+ 2	*	+ 0.5	+ 60	+ 30	+ 350	10
4 + months	+ 0.2	+ 0.5	+ 2	*	+ 0.5	+ 60	+ 30	+ 350	10

* No increment; ** after age 65 the RNI is 10 µg/d for men and women; *** for last trimester only.
[1] Based on protein providing 14.7% of EAR for energy. Crown copyright. Reproduced with the permission of the Controller of The Stationery Office.

Reference Nutrient Intakes for minerals

Age	Calcium mg/d	Phosphorus[1] mg/d	Magnesium mg/d	Sodium[2] mg/d	Potassium[3] mg/d	Chloride[4] mg/d	Iron mg/d	Zinc mg/d	Copper mg/d	Selenium µg/d	Iodine µg/d
0–3 months	525	400	55	210	800	320	1.7	4.0	0.2	10	50
4–6 months	525	400	60	280	850	400	4.3	4.0	0.3	13	60
7–9 months	525	400	75	320	700	500	7.8	5.0	0.3	10	60
10–12 months	525	400	80	350	700	500	7.8	5.0	0.3	10	60
1–3 years	350	270	85	500	800	800	6.9	5.0	0.4	15	70
4–6 years	450	350	120	700	1100	1100	6.1	6.5	0.6	20	100
7–10 years	550	450	200	1200	2000	1800	8.7	7.0	0.7	30	110
Males											
11–14 years	1000	775	280	1600	3100	2500	11.3	9.0	0.8	45	130
15–18 years	1000	775	300	1600	3500	2500	11.3	9.5	1.0	70	140
19–50 years	700	550	300	1600	3500	2500	8.7	9.5	1.2	75	140
50 + years	700	550	300	1600	3500	2500	8.7	9.5	1.2	75	140
Females											
11–14 years	800	625	280	1600	3100	2500	14.8[5]	9.0	0.8	45	130
15–18 years	800	625	300	1600	3500	2500	14.8[5]	7.0	1.0	60	140
19–50 years	700	550	270	1600	3500	2500	14.8[5]	7.0	1.2	60	140
50 + years	700	550	270	1600	3500	2500	8.7	7.0	1.2	60	140
Pregnancy	*	*	*	*	*	*	*	*	*	*	*
Lactation:											
0–4 months	+ 550	+ 440	+ 50	*	*	*	*	+ 6.0	+ 0.3	+ 15	*
4 + months	+ 550	+ 440	+ 50	*	*	*	*	+ 2.5	+ 0.3	+ 15	*

* No increment.

[1] Phosphorus RNI is set equal to calcium in molar terms.

[2] 1 mmol sodium = 23 mg.

[3] 1 mmol potassium = 39 mg.

[4] Corresponds to sodium 1 mmol = 35.5 mg.

[5] Insufficient for women with high menstrual losses where the most practical way of meeting iron requirements is to take iron supplements.

Crown copyright. Reproduced with the permission of the Controller of The Stationery Office.

Safet intakes

Nutrient	Safe intake
Vitamins	
Pantothenic acid	–
adults	3–7 mg/d
infants	1.7 mg/d
Biotin	10–200 µg/d
Vitamin E	
men	above 4 mg/d
women	above 3 mg/d
infants	0.4 mg/g polyunsaturated fatty acids
Vitamin K	
adults	1 µg/kg/d
infants	10 µg/d
Minerals	
Manganese	
adults	1.4 mg (26 µmol)/d
infants and children	16 µg (0.3 µmol)/d
Molybdenum	–
adults	50–400 µg/d
infants, children and adolescents	0.5–1.5 µg/kg/d
Chromium	
adults	25 µg (0.5 µmol)/d
children and adolescents	0.1–1.0 µg (2–20 µmol)/kg/d
Fluoride (for infants only)	0.05 mg (3 µmol)/kg/d

Appendix 2
Functions, Food Sources and Deficiency Symptoms of Vitamins, Minerals and Trace Elements

Vitamins: main functions and food sources

Vitamin	Main function	Main food sources	Possible symptoms of deficiency
Fat soluble			
A (retinol)	Health of mucosal membranes; growth; colour and night vision	Liver, kidney, dairy products, eggs, fortified margarine, butter, fish liver oils	Night blindness (rare); dryness of conjunctiva and cornea; increased frequency of infections
Beta-carotene	Anti-oxidant	Dark green leafy vegetables, carrots, peaches, apricots, cantaloupe melon	Possible role in cancer
D (calciferol; cholecalciferol, ergocalciferol)	Growth and development of bones and teeth by regulating calcium metabolism	Oily fish, fortified margarine, butter, eggs, fish liver oils, fortified breakfast cereals; action of ultraviolet light on skin	Rickets and osteomalacia (see Chapter 13)
E (alpha-tocopherol)	Anti-oxidant; protects cells from free radical damage	Wholegrain cereals, wheatgerm, vegetables, eggs, nuts, peanut butter	No definable syndrome
K (menaphthone)	Blood clotting; energy metabolism	Green leafy vegetables, fruit, nuts, wholegrain cereals	Prolonged clotting time; tendency to bleed
Water soluble			
B₁ (thiamin)	Energy metabolism, particularly carbohydrate	Bread, wholegrain cereals, fortified breakfast cereals, yeast extract, pulses, nuts, pork, liver	Anorexia, weakness, headache, tachycardia (early symptoms); beri-beri; Wernicke's encephalopathy and Korsakoff's psychosis (seen in alcoholism)
B₂ (riboflavin)	Energy metabolism, particularly fat and protein	Milk and dairy products, fortified breakfast cereals, yeast extract, meat, green vegetables	Angular stomatitis, soreness of lips and tongue, seborrhoeic dermatitis, cheilosis
Niacin (nicotinamide, nicotinic acid)	Energy metabolism	Meat, fish, nuts, fortified breakfast cereals, yeast extract, wholemeal bread	Vague – decreased appetite and weight weakness, irritability, inability to concentrate, abdominal discomfort, Pellegra (diarrhoea, dementia, dermatitis)

Cont.

Vitamins: main functions and food sources cont.

Vitamin	Main function	Main food sources	Possible symptoms of deficiency
B₆ (pyridoxine)	Protein metabolism	Meat, fish, fortified breakfast cereals, pulses, nuts, yeast extract	Vague – dermatitis, glossitis, stomatitis
B₁₂ (cyanocobalamin)	Red blood cell production: important for health of nervous system	Meat, fish, eggs, milk, cheese, fortified yeast extract, fortified breakfast cereals	Risk in vegans (see Chapter 21). Megaloblastic anaemia, neuropathy, infertility in females, sore tongue, tingling of extremities. Pernicious anaemia (see Chapter 10)
Folate (folic acid)	Red blood cell production; important for health of nervous system	Liver and kidney, wholegrain cereals, pulses, green vegetables, yeast extract	Possible role in neural tube defects (see Chapter 15) Megaloblastic anaemia (see Chapter 10)
Biotin	Protein and fat metabolism	Liver and kidney, eggs, fish, pulses, vegetables	Very rare. Loss of appetite; affects growth
Pantothenic acid	Energy metabolism	Meat, milk, eggs, cereals, pulses	Very rare. Tingling in hands and feet, fatigue, cramp
C (ascorbic acid)	Maintenance of all tissues; wound healing; antioxidant	Citrus fruit, fruit juice, berries, potatoes, green vegetables	Scurvy (risk in elderly). Malaise, weakness, pain in joints and bones (due to haemorrhage), swollen and bleeding gums, poor wound healing

Minerals and trace elements: main functions and food sources

Mineral or trace element	Main functions	Main food sources	Possible symptoms of deficiency
Mineral			
Calcium	Growth and development of bones and teeth; blood clotting; nerve and muscle function	Milk, cheese, yoghurt, canned fish, bread, nuts, green vegetables	Possible acceleration of osteoporosis
Magnesium	Energy metabolism; muscle function	Green vegetables, wholegrain cereals	Apathy and muscle weakness
Phosphorus	Energy metabolism; strength and support for bones and teeth; cell membrane function, contractility	Meat, milk, dairy products, nuts, yeast and cereals	Very unlikely
Potassium	Maintenance of fluid and electrolyte balance; muscle function	Fruit and vegetables, meat, milk and bread	Very unlikely
Sodium	Maintenance of fluid and electrolyte balance; nerve and muscle function	Salt, processed (particularly smoked) meat and fish products, bread, breakfast cereals	Very unlikely
Trace element			
Chromium	Carbohydrate and fat metabolism; co-factor for insulin	Liver and kidney, brewer's yeast, wholegrain cereals	Possibly glucose intolerance
Copper	Component of many enzymes, immune system, growth and formation	Meat, fish, green vegetables, cereals, pulses	Very rare
Fluoride	Contributes to tooth formation	Tea, fish, tap water	Role in tooth decay
Iodine	Thyroid hormone formation	Seafood, cereals, vegetables and meat	Thyroid disorders

Cont.

Minerals and trace elements: main functions and food sources

Mineral or trace element	Main functions	Main food sources	Possible symptoms of deficiency
Iron	Red blood cell formation; enzym reactions	Liver and kidney, meat, corned beef, fortified breakfast cereals, green vegetables	Anaemia (see Chapter 10) Mild disease – fatigue, weakness, gastrointestinal disturbance Severe anaemia – breathing difficulty, heart failure, angina
Manganese	Component of enzymes	Green vegetables, nuts, pulses, wholegrain cereals	Weight loss, skeletal abnormalities, convulsions
Molybdenum	Component of enzymes	Vegetables, pulses, wholegrain cereals	Unknown
Selenium	Anti-oxidant – acts with vitamin E to prevent cell damage	Cereals, nuts, kidney, liver, meat, milk, eggs	Possible role in cancer and CHD
Zinc	Tissue repair and wound healing, enzyme reactions, taste; immune system	Meat, shellfish, milk, dairy products, cereals, nuts	Skin rash, hair loss, poor wound healing, impaired taste

Appendix 3
Dietary Sources of Iron

Food portion	Iron centre (mg)
Lamb's liver (90 g)	9.0
Red meat, roast (85 g)	2.5
1 beef steak (155 g)	5.4
1 chicken leg (190 g)	1.0
Sardines (70 g)	2.0
1 egg	1.2
Lentils, kidney beans or other pulses (105 g)	2.5
Dhal, chickpea (155 g)	4.8
lentil (155 g)	2.6
1 small can baked beans (225 g)	3.0
2 slices wholemeal bread (70 g)	2.0
2 slices white bread (70 g)	1.0
1 chapatti (70 g)	1.6
Muesli (95 g)	4.0
Bran flakes (45 g)	9.0
Green vegetables (100 g)	0.5
1 small bag peanuts (25 g)	0.5
8 dried apricots (50 g)	2.1
2 handfuls raisins (35 g)	0.6

Dietary Sources of Calcium

Food portion	Calcium content (mg)
1 pint whole milk	700
1 pint semi-skimmed milk	700
1 pint skimmed milk	700
Hard cheese, e.g. Cheddar (50 g)	400
1 carton yoghurt (150 g)	250
Sardines, with bones (70 g)	385
Prawns (80 g)	120
2 slices white bread (70 g)	80
2 slices wholemeal bread (70 g)	40
Lentils, kidney beans or chickpeas (105 g)	40–70
Dhal, chickpea (155 g)	99
1 small can baked beans (225 g)	100
Soya beans (105 g)	90
Tofu (60 g)	300
20 almonds (20 g)	50
1 tablespoon sesame seeds (20 g)	140
Tahini paste on 1 slice bread (10 g)	70
Broccoli (100 g)	75
Spring greens (100 g)	35
1 large orange (250 g)	70

Appendix 5
Dietary Sources of Vitamin D

Food portion	Vitamin D content (µg)
1 pint whole milk	0.18
1 pint semi-skimmed milk	0.06
1 pint fortified skimmed milk (various brands)	0.6–0.12
1 pint goat's milk	0.6
2 tablespoons dried skimmed milk (30 g)	1.0
1 mug Ovaltine	0.7
1 mug Horlicks	0.7
1 mug Build-Up	3.0
1 mug Complan	1.5
Hard cheese, e.g. Cheddar (50 g)	0.1
Feta cheese (50 g)	0.25
1 carton whole milk yoghurt (150 g)	0.06
1 carton low fat yoghurt (150 g)	0.01
1 egg	1.0
Butter on 1 slice bread (10 g)	0.25
Margarine on 1 slice bread (10 g)	2.5
Low-fat spread on 1 slice bread (10 g)	2.5
2 tablespoons ghee (30 g)	0.6
Lamb's liver (90 g)	0.5
Sardines (70 g)	5.6
Tinned salmon (100 g)	12.5
Tinned pilchards (100 g)	8.0
Tinned tuna (100 g)	5.0
1 grilled herring (150 g)	25.0
2 kipper fillets (110 g)	25.0
2 mackerel fillets (110 g)	21.0
2 teaspoons cod liver oil	21.0

Note: Some breakfast cereals are fortified with vitamin D.

Index